THE GROWING FAMILY SERIES

Safe and Healthy

A parent's guide to children's
illnesses and accidents

Safe and Healthy

A Parent's Guide to Children's Illnesses and Accidents

William Sears, M.D.

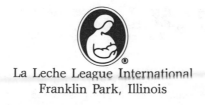

La Leche League International
Franklin Park, Illinois

© 1989 by William Sears, M.D.
All rights reserved
93 92 91 90 89   7 6 5 4 3 2 1

Printed in the United States of America

Photo credits: pages 5, 51, 59, 169, 177, 200, Gwen Gotsch; pages 9, 25,
    29, 37, 44, 67, 82, 95, 107, 111, 115, 125, 158, 218, 224, 231, Dale
    Pfeiffer; pages 12, 192, William Sears; page 184, compliments of Nojo,
    Inc.
Edited by Gwen Gotsch
Illustrations by Tony Yee
Cover design and illustration by Kim Stuffelbeam
Library of Congress Catalog Card Number 89-084859
ISBN 912500-22-0

Dedicated to my family,
Jim, Bob, Peter, Hayden, Erin, Matthew,
Stephen, and Martha

CONTENTS

Chapter 11
First-Aid Procedures for Common Emergencies
and Injuries 203

FOREWORD

Parents watching over the health of their children need both information and reassurance. In SAFE AND HEALTHY: A PARENT'S GUIDE TO CHILDREN'S ILLNESSES AND ACCIDENTS, Dr. William Sears gives parents the information they need to keep their child healthy and offers a variety of suggestions for comforting the child if he does get sick.

Dr. Sears provides specific guidelines for parents to use in determining the seriousness of their child's illness. This will prevent countless sleepless nights and unnecessary worry. He also offers suggestions about when to call the doctor and how to accurately describe the child's illness over the phone. He tells when and why the doctor may want to see your child rather than suggesting treatment by phone.

As in all of his books in the *Growing Family Series,* Dr. Sears extols the benefits of breastfeeding and the value of attachment parenting. He explains that breastfeeding offers immunities and other health benefits that last well beyond infancy. And his commitment to attachment parenting is clear when he describes how knowing your child well helps you recognize symptoms of illness.

One important point in this book may be so subtle that it could be overlooked—the importance of an ongoing relationship between the family and the doctor.

This may not be easy to achieve nowadays with families moving frequently and doctors who share group practices. But when the doctor sees the family members through a variety of situations and has confidence in the parents' capability and commitment to their child, he or she will be more comfortable sending the sick child home to be cared for by parents instead of adding the stress of hospitalization to the situation. Parents should be aware of this as they seek the healthcare professionals they will turn to when illness strikes.

This book is one that every parent will want to have on hand. As I read this book, I couldn't help wishing it had been available when my own four children were growing up. It's the kind of book that gives parents a feeling of confidence in their ability to care for their child. I'm going to make sure my daughter has a copy to read while my grandson is still a toddler.

Judy Torgus
La Leche League International

PREFACE

Child-rearing is anxiety-producing enough when children are well, let alone when they are sick. I hope that this book will take much of the anxiety out of caring for a sick child. By learning to recognize early signs of illness and by knowing what to watch for to determine if an illness is or is not serious, you become more comfortable in parenting your sick child. You will also know when to call your child's doctor and will be able to communicate more effectively with healthcare professionals.

The medical advice I present is based on my experience in nearly 20 years of pediatric practice, as well as my years as a father of seven children. I have also consulted with trusted colleagues and have read the most up-to-date medical literature. The information in this book will help you use the current medical care system. There are also many time-tested self-help remedies to assist you in being your child's "home doctor."

I purposely avoid questionable forms of treatment. Children are too valuable, and parents too vulnerable, for any book to propose treatments which have not been proven safe and effective. (Love for your child makes you vulnerable to any suggestions that promise to help your child feel better.)

Keeping children safe and healthy is a goal parents and healthcare professionals strive for. This book is designed to help you achieve that goal. As in all the books of the *Growing Family Series*, SAFE AND HEALTHY is meant to help you know your child better, to help your child feel right, and ultimately to help you better enjoy your child. If you increase your sensitivity to your well child, you will find it easier to comfort and understand your sick child.

CHAPTER 1

How to Keep Your Child Healthy

Well children are usually a joy to parents. Sick children are less of a joy. A child who feels right is more likely to act right, and a child who acts right is more pleasant to be around. When the child is sick, the whole family may be "sick." Parents of a sick child often tell me, "He's been like a bear all week. He doesn't sleep, he won't eat, and he's irritable all day long. He's driving us crazy."

Children do get sick. This is a fact of life for parents. But you can lessen the chances of your child becoming ill. There are many things you can do to help keep your child healthy.

Developing a Parenting Style That Helps Your Child Stay Healthy

Your parenting style is your way of caring for your child. New parents especially are bombarded with childcare advice from well-meaning friends and relatives. But not all advice—even from experts—is appropriate for all parents

1

and children. You as a parent must find a parenting style that allows both you and your child to thrive and feel right.

During my 20 years in pediatric practice, I have noticed that parenting style affects the health of children. The parenting that I have been most impressed with is what I call **attachment parenting**. The characteristics of this style include:

A close relationship between parent and child, beginning in the newborn period when parents spend lots of time getting to know their baby

Timely responses to an infant's cries (avoiding the "let him cry it out" approach)

Extended breastfeeding with child-led weaning

"Wearing" your baby (carrying him in your arms or a baby carrier) as much as possible

Sharing sleep with your baby by having him sleep in your bed, if this style helps all family members sleep better.

I do not mean to imply that if parents do all of these things they will have children who are always healthy, but on the whole, I believe that this style of parenting will increase your chances of having a healthy child. In making choices about your parenting style, you must take into account your own situation, your lifestyle, and any medical conditions in your child that affect the way you all interact.

How Attachment Parenting Contributes to Wellness
I recently participated in a discussion group with pediatricians, family doctors, and other primary health care physicians. We were discussing what qualities we like to see develop in new parents. Most everyone agreed that responsiveness—the ability of a parent to respond appropriately to the infant or child's cues—was most important. A few dissenters clung to the old theory that responding to babies' and young children's cues will spoil

them. However, when research was presented which demonstrated that responsiveness does not spoil children, even the diehard believers in the spoiling theory were won over.

Attachment parenting promotes responsiveness. It increases the sensitivity between parent and child. The parents are better able to detect when something is wrong with their child, and the child is better able to tell the parents that something is wrong.

Here's how it works. Attachment parenting promotes closeness between parent and child and helps the parent and children to know each other better. It helps you "feel" for each other. As one mother put it, "I know how to read my child." This sensitivity to children underlies statements I hear in my office from concerned mothers:

"I know what my child is like when she's well, and I know she's not feeling well now."

"I don't know what's wrong, but my baby's acting differently and I'm worried."

"I know his cries. These are not just upset cries, he hurts somewhere."

Attachment parenting makes the parent's powers of observation more acute.

This style of parenting also causes biological changes in a mother. Breastfeeding, one of the elements of attachment parenting, causes mothers to have higher levels of prolactin. As a father of seven and a pediatrician for 20 years, I can honestly say that I do not understand the effects of this hormone, but I have grown to respect it. I often refer to it as the "sensitivity hormone." Prolactin seems to me like some magical substance that tells mothers just what their babies are thinking and feeling.

Breastfeeding mothers seem to develop an acute awareness of changes in their babies' behavior which may signal the onset of an illness. Two mothers have given me some tips on early detection of ear infections in tiny infants. One mother related that she can always tell that her baby is developing an ear infection by a change in the baby's sucking patterns. Another mother suspected her one-month-old baby girl had an ear infection because she did not want to put her head down to nurse on one side, although she nursed well on the other side. Babies' ears hurt more when lying with the affected ear down.

How about the child's sensitivity to the parent? When parents use the attachment style, a child becomes accustomed to having his signals read and his cues responded to. This motivates him to develop a higher level of communication with the parents because he knows that they will understand him. A magnificent language of mutual sensitivity develops between a parent and a child when they are closely attached to one another.

Attachment Parenting Benefits the Doctor
Take the example of a nine-month-old infant brought into my office because of a fever. (This happens almost daily.) I examine the child to try to determine if whatever is going on is something to worry about. Over the years I have noticed that infants and children of attachment-style parents radiate an atmosphere of trust that is most noticeable when they are ill. They generally trust the examining physician and protest less during an examination. It is as if there were some inner signal from parent to child, telling him that this person who is putting a stick in his mouth, shining a light in his ears, and poking at his tummy is actually doing all this to help. An infant who is easier to examine actually helps the doctor make a more accurate diagnosis.

Not only does attachment parenting make it easier to examine a child; it also makes me feel more secure about the parent's ability to care for a sick child. Many childhood illnesses, quite honestly, fall into the category "I don't know what's wrong, so let's wait and see what develops." Does this nine-month-old infant with a fever have an underlying infection that I'm not yet able to diagnose, or is this just a passing virus? Time and changing symptoms will tell. I may say to the parents, "At this point,

I feel that your child has a viral illness that isn't serious. He should improve within a few days, but please get in touch with me right away if any worrisome signs or changes occur." I tell them what to watch for, but in reality, I am relying on the parent's own powers of observation and intuition to recognize if the child's condition worsens. It is almost as if I am releasing the child to another set of doctors. But what are the credentials of these "doctors"? Will these parents really be able to tell if their child is getting worse instead of better? What comfort there is when I entrust a child into the hands of parents who have practiced attachment parenting! I know that they know their child, that they will recognize any worrisome changes, and that they will call me if their child worsens.

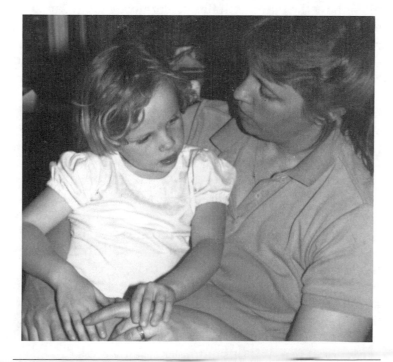

Knowing your child when she is well will make you more sensitive to her when she is ill.

Attachment Parenting Makes Comforting Easier
During the early years parents spend many hours comforting children who are sick. Parents who have practiced the attachment style of parenting are generally better able to comfort their child, and the child is more easily comforted. The overwhelming sensitivity between parent and child increases the parent's repertoire of comforting measures. These parents have already had lots of practice with walking, holding, nursing, touching, and massaging a crying or distressed baby. The child, in turn, has built such a trusting relationship with his parents that he surrenders easily to their soothing.

This is especially true during critical illnesses when children are hospitalized. I frequently impress upon parents that they are a very important part of the team of professionals taking care of their child. Here's an example of how the parent's ability to comfort a child can have an amazing effect. I had to hospitalize Tony, a fourteen-month-old infant who had severe croup. As Tony's condition worsened, his airway became more obstructed, and he had more and more difficulty breathing. (This generally happens when a child with croup becomes increasingly worried and anxious and cannot be comforted.) It was starting to look as if we might have to place a tube in his windpipe to help him breathe, a procedure which is very traumatic but potentially life-saving. I told Tony's mother that we would have to do this if Tony didn't settle down a bit and relax his airway. She asked if she could try helping Tony relax so that we could avoid this emergency procedure. I agreed. Over the next five minutes this mother took charge of her infant and used all the maternal comforting measures that she had so repeatedly rehearsed in the first months of Tony's life. (Tony had been a colicky, high-need baby who needed constant comforting.) Tony relaxed, as did his airway. Emergency intubation was not necessary, and Tony soon went on to full recovery. It was as if this mother herself were a therapeutic intervention. She plugged herself into her child and with her comforting measures allowed calm to flow from herself into her child.

Pediatric intensive care specialists have long recognized the therapeutic value of a parent's touch. Low birthweight babies grow better, children heal faster, and hospital stays are shortened when the pediatric patient is given high doses of nurturing care by the parent. (See references at the end of the chapter for a discussion of the scientific basis of how attachment parenting affects health.)

How Good Nutrition Contributes to Good Health

The Effects of Breastfeeding

Breast milk may be considered your baby's first immunization. Human milk, like blood, contains many elements which help your infant fight against infection. Because human milk is a living tissue, it contains a rich supply of white blood cells which fight against germs in your baby's intestines.

Human milk also contains a large supply of special disease-fighting proteins called immunoglobulins. While your baby was in the womb he received maternal immunoglobulins through the placenta. These immunoglobulins help to protect your baby from disease during his first months of life, but they slowly disappear and by nine months are mostly gone. As these maternal immunoglobulins are disappearing your baby begins to manufacture his own, but in the early months he makes them very slowly. Breast milk provides immunoglobulins at the very time when an infant is most susceptible to illness. In fact, human milk is highest in disease-fighting properties during the newborn period, when babies are most susceptible to infection. Some of these immunoglobulins act like a protective paint and coat the inside of the intestines, preventing the growth of unfavorable bacteria.

Human milk also contains elements called resistance factors which have antibacterial and antiviral properties and also contribute to the growth of favorable bacteria in the intestines. The intestines of breastfed babies are colonized by more friendly bacteria, such as the organism *Lactobacillus bifidus*. This organism helps crowd out the growth of other bacteria and makes the environment in the intestines less favorable for the growth of harmful bacteria. Other friendly bacteria also help to keep harmful germs in check and aid in the production of certain beneficial nutrients. In medical terms, we say that breastfed infants have healthier intestinal flora. Because the intestines of breastfed infants are colonized with more friendly bacteria, diarrheal disease (gastroenteritis) is less frequent and less severe in breastfed infants. Recent discoveries have shown that properties in breast milk help intestinal germs to go through mutations that make them less harmful. A mother's milk has been found to have therapeutic properties in treating intestinal infections in her baby. I have noticed that during flu epidemics breastfed infants get fewer illnesses, and if they do get sick, they recover sooner. In fact, it is usually wise to encourage a mother to continue breastfeeding if her baby has an intestinal infection.

It is particularly exciting to see how human milk provides ongoing protection against unwanted intestinal germs. If a new germ enters a mother's body, she produces antibodies to this germ. These antibodies are delivered to the infant through her milk, thus protecting her baby from the same germ. Since mother and baby are, most likely, exposed to the same germs, the mother, by breastfeeding, helps to defend her baby against the germs in his environment.

Breastfeeding also indirectly contributes to health by lessening allergies. Allergy to cow's milk and dairy products is a common contributing factor to respiratory and gastrointestinal illnesses in children in the first few years. In the early weeks of a child's life the intestines may allow potential allergens to pass through to the bloodstream where they can set up an allergic reaction. Human milk has certain elements which act like a protective paint, coating the intestines and preventing the potential allergens from getting through. Instead of being overwhelmed by food allergens in cow's milk formula in the first weeks of life, the breastfed baby's immune system is exposed to only the small amounts of food proteins that may appear in his mother's milk. This allows a child to gradually build up his acceptance of most foods.

Benefits of extended breastfeeding. Not only does breastfeeding contribute to the overall general health of the infant, but extended breastfeeding, well into the second year or even longer, is also advisable. I have noticed that nursing toddlers are more trusting and therefore easier to examine during an illness. Nursing toddlers who are vomiting or have diarrhea can usually tolerate breast milk, and will nurse frequently while they are ill. This lessens the risk of becoming dehydrated and needing hospitalization. Breast milk also provides important nutritional elements, especially for children who are allergic to dairy products. These and other reasons are why I have a sign in my office saying "Early weaning not recommended for infants."

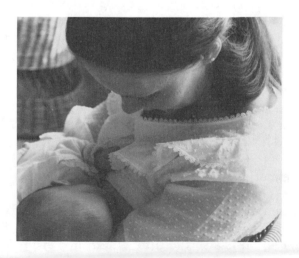

Breastfeeding helps babies stay healthy.

Good Food and Good Health

Good nutrition in general promotes good health both in children and adults. Children who are undernourished become debilitated. Sufficient amounts of protein, vitamins, and calories in your child's diet increase his ability to fight infection. Children with insufficient iron in their diet have low amounts of hemoglobin in their blood, a condition called anemia. Anemic children are more prone to infections. Iron-rich foods include: breast milk (the iron in human milk is absorbed better than the iron found in any other food), fish, beef, cereal, meats, and red beans. Dairy products and most vegetables are poor sources of iron. If your child does have a poor diet (or is the classic "picky eater"), your doctor may recommend supplemental vitamins.

Keeping Germs Away

Germs are about the only things that children seem to share easily. During the first two or three years, as children are building up their immunity, they are especially vulnerable to infection. The more they are exposed to crowds of other children, the more infections they will have. We don't live in an ideal world, and it is unrealistic to expect the child to grow up in a protective bubble. But here are some suggestions to decrease your child's risk of getting sick.

Avoid crowded day care as much as possible. If day care is absolutely necessary in your own family situation, try for a situation in which a small number of children are cared for in a home and the day care provider is very careful to screen sick children. If your child is in day care and is experiencing lots of respiratory and intestinal infections, change his day care situation.

Church nurseries contribute to the sharing of germs. The times in their lives when children are most disruptive in church is also the time when they are most susceptible to contagious illnesses. If your young child or his siblings have any signs of contagious illness (fever, runny nose, diarrhea, productive cough), then keep him out of the nursery.

Watch your child's playmates for potentially contagious diseases, especially if your child has a history of frequent respiratory and/or intestinal illnesses. Keep your child away from playmates who have signs of contagious illness. Children are most contagious the day before and the first few days of a respiratory or intestinal illness. A child who has had a cold for a week or two is probably no longer contagious.

Other Environmental Contributors to Disease

Exposure of a child to cigarette smoke is a very common yet grossly underestimated cause of illness. It has been documented that children of parents who smoke have three times the number of doctor visits, primarily for respiratory illnesses and ear infections. Smoke is an irritant that contributes to stuffy noses and retained nasal secretions. Retained secretions in the nose, breathing passages, and ears are good places for bacteria to grow and start respiratory infections. Any environmental pollutant (smoke, perfumes, hair sprays, exhaust fumes, construction dust from house remodeling) can increase the incidence of respiratory infections in children.

Well Child Exams and Immunizations

Another way to help keep your child healthy is to follow your doctor's schedule for well baby and well child exams. In my office we use this schedule:

Monthly for the first six months

Every three months from six to eighteen months

Every six months from eighteen months to three years

Yearly thereafter.

The frequency of these exams may change depending upon the number of children in your family and the overall health of your child.

Well baby and child exams provide a number of benefits. During these exams your doctor will discuss various aspects of preventive medicine such as nutrition, hygiene, immunizations, and ways to avoid contagious diseases. Your doctor will also tell you how to recognize signs of illness in your child and provide education on childhood safety and accident prevention. Well child exams also act as a reference point for illness. Your doctor can make a much more accurate diagnosis when your child is sick if he or she has become acquainted with your child when he is well. I find myself at a disadvantage when I must treat a child for an illness when I haven't seen the child and parents previously for periodic checkups. During these scheduled exams your doctor increases his or her knowledge of your child and of you as parents. Exams also help you get to know your doctor, so that you will feel more comfortable seeking medical help when your child is ill. Check-ups are a wise investment in your child's health.

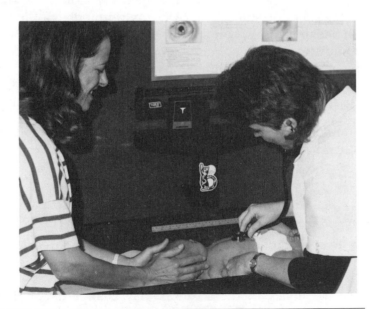

Well baby exams benefit both mother and baby.

What about Immunizations?

Immunizations have received a lot of bad press lately. Unfortunately this has done more to confuse the public than to educate it. Parents, wanting to do what is best for their child, are often caught in a dilemma. They worry that if they have their child immunized, he may experience a bad reaction; if their child is not immunized, they worry that he will get the disease itself.

Today's parents do not remember the pre-vaccine era, when infectious diseases seriously harmed the health of children. I can still remember as a young child seeing or reading about other children spending years in iron lungs for treatment of polio. As a young intern in pediatrics I heard the coughing and choking of very uncomfortable infants on the whooping cough ward—infants who had not been immunized. I remember the encephalitis caused by measles and the birth defects in babies of mothers who had German measles during pregnancy. These diseases are not common anymore, perhaps because of the vaccines.

Immunizations stimulate your child's immunologic defenses to produce antibodies against the germ that causes a particular illness. A vaccine is made from a part of the germ itself or from a germ changed in such a way that it does not cause disease but nevertheless stimulates the body to react as if it were the real thing. If the real germ enters the body, the antibodies produced by the vaccine will be able to fight the germ and no disease or a milder disease will result.

Every vaccine (and, in fact, any substance that is put into a child's body, be it a medicine or a food) has both risks and benefits. When evaluating a vaccine we try to determine what is the risk/benefit ratio. If the risks of a reaction to a vaccine are worse than the risks from the disease that the vaccine is designed to prevent, then the vaccine has a high risk-to-benefit ratio and is not a safe vaccine. An example of this is the current thinking on the smallpox vaccine. Many years ago the risk of death or serious illness from smallpox was much higher than the risks associated with the vaccine. Vaccination against smallpox was practiced around the world, and it was difficult to escape the familiar scratch and scar on the upper arm. The smallpox vaccine initially had a low risk/benefit ratio. However, the worldwide vaccination program was so effective that nowadays smallpox has been nearly eradicated. The risks associated with the vaccine outweigh the extremely small risk of contracting the disease, so routine smallpox vaccination has been discontinued.

There are currently eight vaccines in common use. These are vaccines for diphtheria, pertussis (whooping cough), tetanus, measles, mumps, rubella (German measles), polio, and the newer Hib vaccine (for the bacteria *Hemophilus influenzae* type B, a common cause of respiratory infections and meningitis in young children). Diphtheria, pertussis, and tetanus are usually given together in a DPT shot; measles, mumps, and rubella are combined in the MMR. The polio vaccine is given orally. All of these vaccines have a low risk/benefit ratio.

However, the pertussis vaccine has been a cause of increasing concern. Of all the vaccines it is the least effective in preventing the disease it is designed to combat, and it presents the greatest risk of serious reactions. The media, along with concerned parents and healthcare professionals, have called attention to the fact that the whooping cough vaccine is not a very good vaccine. This has stimulated researchers and manufacturers to work on a safer and more effective vaccine, which will probably be available within a few years. Countries which have temporarily stopped the routine use of the pertussis vaccine have encountered whooping cough epidemics shortly thereafter and have therefore resumed routine vaccination for whooping cough.

Unfortunately the concerns about the whooping cough vaccine have carried over to other vaccines and have created a lot of fear about other vaccines as well. As a result some parents (still the minority), wishing to do what they feel is best, have withheld all immunizations from their child. This is unfortunate.

My personal opinion, at this writing, is that children should be immunized according to the dosage and schedule recommended by the Committee on Infectious Diseases of the American Academy of Pediatrics (see chart), unless special medical circumstances are present. The immunization schedule should be followed as closely as possible. The initial series of three DPT vaccines may be given as closely as one month apart. Interrupting the recommended schedule does not interfere with the development of immunity; it is not necessary to start the series again, regardless of the time elapsed. It is not necessary to delay your child's immunizations if he has a cold. Immunizations should not be given while your child is generally sick or is running a fever, but immunizations need not be delayed because of a common cold. There are special health considerations which may prompt your doctor to alter the schedule and dosage of your child's immunizations.

Parents who are still uncomfortable about following this schedule should consider a number of factors in making a decision about immunizations. Do you live in a high-risk area of the country (e.g., New York, Florida, Texas, and California) where there is a large influx of unimmunized persons? This increases the likelihood of your child's being exposed to the diseases prevented by immu-

Immunization Schedule

Age	Vaccine
2 mos	DPT, oral polio
4 mos	DPT, oral polio
6 mos	DPT, oral polio (optional)
1 year	Tuberculin test
15 mos	Measles, mumps, rubella (MMR)
18 mos-2 years	Hib, DPT
4-5 years	DPT

nizations. I believe that full immunization is wise in these circumstances. If you live in a relatively low-risk area and your child is not in day care or exposed to a lot of other children, perhaps the pertussis vaccine could be omitted.

Some parents who are uncertain about the whooping cough vaccine decide to have their children receive it later in childhood. This is unwise. Whooping cough is most serious in the first year of life, when it can be fatal to a tiny infant. Whooping cough becomes less serious as the child matures, and the six weeks of coughing it produces may be no more than a nuisance for the older child. If you are going to immunize your child against pertussis, it is wisest to do so at the time in his life when contacting the illness will be most detrimental. Parents with reservations about the whooping cough vaccine may elect to receive the initial series (at two, four, and six months of age) and omit the pertussis vaccine at eighteen months and school entry. In my opinion this is not an unwise choice since the seriousness of the illness decreases with age while the reaction rate may increase.

Although rubella itself is not a serious disease, it is very important that all children receive rubella immunizations. The vaccine is given as a public health measure. A rubella infection during pregnancy can cause birth defects, and the immunization is given to prevent children with rubella from transmitting it to pregnant women. If there were no vaccine for rubella, approximately eighty-five percent of women of childbearing age would be immune to the disease anyway, because they contracted it as children and hence, have developed immunities to it. Therefore, the "natural" immunization program would be eighty-five percent effective. If only fifty percent of children are given the vaccine, the incidence of rubella in children would decline significantly, even among children who are not immunized, since they would be much less likely to come into contact with another child who has rubella. Therefore, these unimmunized children would reach adulthood without becoming immune to rubella, since they neither received the vaccine nor developed natural immunity after having the disease. This would leave a higher percent-age of childbearing women vulnerable to rubella infec-tion during pregnancy than if there were no vaccination program at all. This is why some public health researchers feel that rubella immunization should be an "all or none" program: either no person should receive the vaccine, or all persons should be vaccinated. If only some persons are vaccinated, the result may be worse than if the vac-cine is not used at all. In deciding whether to give your child the rubella vaccine, consider first your responsibil-ity to childbearing women and their unborn babies.

There is a theoretical consideration that the immunity conferred by vaccines may wear off in late childhood and adulthood, leaving the individual susceptible to illness later on. Time has not shown this to be the case. At this writing the vaccines in common usage today have been shown to confer at least twenty to thirty years of immu-nity. In the worst case, if immunity should wear off, all that is needed is a booster shot.

What about vaccine reactions?   Any medicine has side effects—undesirable, uncomfortable, and sometimes damaging to the body. This is true of vaccines as well. Reactions to vaccines usually occur within minutes or hours of the injection, except in the case of the MMR vac-cine where reactions occur one to two weeks later. Un-desirable reactions to vaccines depend on your child's own immune response to that vaccine. They are not the fault of the person administering the vaccine. Parents have a right to informed consent; ask your doctor or health care professional about the potential risks of vaccines. If your child does have a reaction to a vaccine, be sure to report the severity of the reaction to your doctor so that your child's future immunization program can be modified.

Pertussis (the P of the DPT) has the highest reaction rate. Exact statistics are difficult to come by. Possibly fifty percent of children have minor discomforts consisting of a slightly sore muscle at the injection site, a generalized achy feeling, and a low-grade fever. These symptoms usually subside within a few hours. Approximately 1 in 300,000 children (again, accurate statistics are hard to come by) will have a severe reaction to the pertussis vaccine, leading to brain damage of varying degrees of severity.

The reason that statistics are hard to come by is that some illnesses that are attributed to reactions to the pertussis vaccine may in fact have been coincidental. In other words, the child would have experienced the illness even if he had not received the DPT shot; the two events just happened to coincide. An example of this is the erroneous but alarming linkage of sudden infant death syndrome (SIDS) with the DPT vaccine. Statistical analysis of the data has failed to show a valid correlation. In one case of SIDS which occurred in my practice, the infant died early in the morning about three hours before the doctor's appointment at which he would have received his first DPT shot. Had the SIDS occurred later in the day, it would have been easy to blame the DPT shot, although the two events happening on the same day was, in fact, only a coincidence.

MMR vaccine may produce reactions in approximately five percent of infants. Reactions occur one to two weeks following the injection of the vaccine and usually consist of three days of varying degrees of fever and a generally sick child. These symptoms subside without harming the child. The rubella vaccine may produce transient joint pain in approximately five percent of infants. The new Hib vaccine may produce transient fever in one or two percent of infants. Reactions to the diphtheria and tetanus vaccines are negligible.

Out of millions of persons receiving the oral polio vaccine, there have been approximately three cases of adults contracting polio presumably from caring for an infant shortly after that infant received an oral polio vaccine. To my knowledge there have been no cases of infants getting polio from the oral polio vaccine. Breastfeeding will not interfere with the effectiveness of the oral polio vaccine.

The list of vaccines needed when traveling to foreign countries changes continually because of outbreaks of various communicable diseases in different parts of the world. Contact your local health department for information about immunizations for the countries you plan to visit. Be sure to carry a stamped immunization card, which states that you have received the required vaccines. It may be required to re-enter your home nation. Immunizations usually required for foreign countries include cholera, yellow fever, and typhoid. You should also receive gamma globulin protection against hepatitis and medication for prevention of malaria.

References
Sears, William. *Nighttime Parenting*. Franklin Park, Illinois: La Leche League International, 1985.
Sears, William. *The Fussy Baby*. Franklin Park, Illinois: La Leche League International, 1985.

CHAPTER 2

General Self-Help Remedies

How often have you heard the advice, "Get plenty of rest, get lots of fluids, take two aspirins, and call me in the morning if you don't feel better"? It may sound like a cliche, a way for a doctor to get off the phone and get back to sleep, but this advice is time-tested and often does the trick. These suggestions, as well as many other gentle ways of caring for your child, can help keep her comfortable during an illness.

How to Recognize When Your Child Is Sick

One of the best ways of being able to recognize that your child is ill is to really know your child when she is well. You can do this by developing a parenting style that helps you really get to know your well child and read her signals. Like the red lights on an automobile dashboard that come on when something is wrong with the engine, the body has its own signals of malfunction. Parents need to learn what they are and how to read them. This is particularly true in infants and young children, who may not always be able to tell you where they hurt.

Fever is the most common sign that tells you a child is sick. Fever is a sign of an underlying illness, not an illness in itself, and needs to be understood in the context of other symptoms and the overall sickness level of the child. A higher fever does not necessarily mean a sicker child. Some non-serious viruses can produce a very high fever; some very serious bacteria are associated with a low fever. Fever that see-saws up and down and is easily controlled by fever-lowering medicines is of much less concern than a fever that stays high and is difficult to bring down. (See Chapter Four for information on treating fever.)

Peaked (pronounced *peak'ed*) is a term you will not find in any medical books. It's an old word that describes the facial appearance of a sick child: puffy, droopy eyes, pale skin, unhappy expression, and the loss of the sparkle that you see on the face of a healthy child. When your child looks peaked, she probably isn't feeling very well.

A mild degree of **lethargy** is common with most childhood illnesses. A child who is lethargic lacks energy and is sluggish. The body needs to become inactive in order to direct energy away from activity and into healing. Severe lethargy produces drowsiness and deep sleep from which it is difficult to arouse a child. Lethargy which progresses into decreasing levels of consciousness— "my child doesn't seem quite with it" —is a cause of great concern. When telling your doctor that your child seems lethargic, always describe just how lethargic she is.

Behavior changes such as irritability and crankiness are common with most childhood illnesses. A child who doesn't feel well doesn't act well. When describing an illness to your doctor always try to assess how much your child is bothered by her symptoms. If she seems generally happy, not much different from her usual self, then there's seldom a serious illness. Some children have a high tolerance for pain and illness and do not act as sick as they really are. In time you will get to know how your child tolerates illness.

Rapid breathing and rapid heartbeat often accompany illness, especially with a fever. This is the body's way of releasing the heat that is generated by the fever. The fast heartbeat and fast breathing usually lessen as the fever is brought down. Continued rapid heartbeat and rapid respirations even after the fever is brought down are worrisome signs and should be reported to your doctor.

Gastrointestinal symptoms (vomiting and/or diarrhea) often accompany childhood illnesses, even though the germ may not be having a direct effect on the intestines. Vomiting commonly accompanies severe ear infections, pneumonia, and severe coughs. Persistent vomiting in a child who is very sick is a worrisome sign, whereas occasional vomiting is not.

How to Help Your Child Feel Better

Rest

During an illness the child's body needs to divert the energy that is usually consumed in physical play into the process of healing. Rest slows down the child's metabolism and frees up energy to help fight the illness. Body parts that hurt—achy heads and tummies, congested chests—don't like to be jostled around. Rest settles painful parts of the body.

Fortunately, children are often better at resting than adults, who are driven by social and economic pressures which may not allow them to rest. It is often not necessary to "make" a child stay in bed. She will usually want to rest the part that hurts and will do so automatically. Young children seldom fake illnesses, nor do they try to cover up when they hurt.

Sometimes it is necessary to use a little parental ingenuity to encourage a child to take it easy. Here are some tips:

Watch television, preferably long children's movies.

Read stories.

Give the child a prolonged back rub.

Encourage the child to tell you a long story.

These tips help to distract the child and take her attention away from the discomfort of her illness. If the child has difficulty sleeping, a mild sedative is often helpful, but a long, drawn-out, not-too-interesting story by mom or dad will often lull the child to sleep. Sometimes tape recordings of children's stories will also do the trick.

TLC
Large doses of tender loving care (TLC) are certainly necessary to parent children through illness. Just like adults, children love special attention when they are sick. It is a good time for special treats, back rubs, soothing words, sympathy, favorite foods—things that say to the sick child, you are a special person with a special need and everybody in the family cares about you. Mental discomfort accompanies every physical illness. TLC helps the child's mind feel good; this can carry over into overall feelings of well-being.

Fresh Air
It is seldom necessary or advisable to keep a child indoors during an illness. Fresh air is therapeutic, both physically and mentally. Dry, stuffy air (especially during winter) usually aggravates respiratory illnesses. Resting outside, or at least in a well-ventilated room, improves a child's mental reaction to her illness. There is something uplifting about the wide open space and fresh air of the outdoors. Reassure grandmother that your child did not get sick in the first place because you took her outdoors and

that she will not get sicker if you take her outdoors before she is well.

Fluids

During most illnesses a child's body loses extra fluid. Fever causes sweating and increased water loss from rapid breathing. Coughing, sneezing, vomiting, and diarrhea are also avenues of increased fluid loss. Dehydration (loss of body fluid) causes an overall unwell feeling which further aggravates the discomfort of the illness. Children usually lose their appetite during an illness and do not want to eat. But they *must* drink, as a general rule, at least twice as much as usual. Home-made popsicles, diluted apple juice, ginger ale, and nutritious juice popsicles are good choices. The "sips and chips" method (small sips of fluids, popsicles, and ice chips) is the best way to encourage a sick child to down lots of fluids. Large volumes of fluids taken too fast may come right back up.

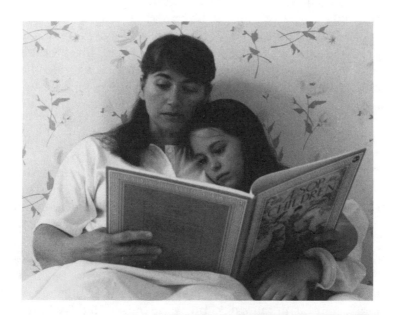

A quiet story helps a child rest.

Feeding the Sick Child

Children often don't want to eat when they're sick, especially with gastrointestinal illnesses. In general, it is more important to drink fluids than to eat. However, it is important that children have adequate calories to fuel the increased demands for energy during an illness. High fever especially causes the body to expend more energy. Protein is needed to heal damaged tissues.

Smaller, frequent feedings work best; in other words, half as much twice as often. Smoothies made with fruit juice, sherbet, protein powder, yogurt, and pureed fresh fruit are a very nutritious and well-tolerated food for the sick child. The child can sip this through a straw at a slow pace. Fruit and honey are particularly good sources of energy for a sick child. Children are prone to having low blood sugar, especially when a diminished appetite is combined with the increased energy demands of illness. This can be a real double whammy for a sick child. Fructose types of sugars (fruit, fruit concentrate, honey) are good sources of steady energy. Soup (preferably homemade broth with chunks of vegetables and chicken) is appreciated and well tolerated by the ill child. (I remember once reading a semi-scientific study that concluded that chicken soup really does help the common cold, although the researchers felt that the benefits came more from the steam than from the soup itself.)

Pain Relievers

Pain relievers are called analgesics. Aspirin, the oldest analgesic, has gradually fallen into disuse in pediatrics because of the possible side effects. Although it has not been conclusively proven, research has linked the taking of aspirin during chicken pox or influenza with a greater risk of developing Reye's syndrome, a serious encephalitis-like disease. Most experts recommend that aspirin not be given to children with a fever. Acetaminophen is almost as effective and is much safer, but aspirin is a slightly better pain reliever. It is wise to check with your doctor about which is better and safer for your child's particular illness.

The directions on most packages of acetaminophen or aspirin state that you should consult your doctor for the proper dosage in children under two years of age. See the chart on page 57 for information about acetaminophen dosage for young children. Note that you can calculate the exact dosage required using the child's weight. I have found that the analgesic dosages listed on the package are too low for many children. Consult your doctor if standard dosages do not seem to relieve your child's discomfort.

Narcotic pain relievers are seldom used in children because of their unpredictable side effects. Codeine, for example, may be prescribed by your doctor in particularly painful illnesses (such as ear infections). While codeine is a more effective analgesic than aspirin or acetaminophen, many children develop allergic reactions or bizarre behavior on codeine. It should be used with caution and only under medical supervision.

Giving Medicines

As Mary Poppins knew, "a spoonful of sugar makes the medicine go down." Sometimes it takes a lot of ingenuity to get children to take their medicine. Here are some points to remember when giving your child medication.

Follow instructions. Be sure you understand your doctor's instructions about giving medicine. Ask questions when your doctor prescribes a medication: How much? How often? At what time of day? Before or after meals? Should I wake my child to give her medicine? What should I do if we inadvertently miss a dose? If the instructions on the medicine bottle differ from what your doctor or pharmacist told you, call your doctor for clarification. If you're confused about the dosage or instructions, call your doctor.

Never use a medicine past the expiration date listed on the package, without first consulting your doctor. The medicine is unlikely to be harmful, but it may not be effective.

Measure carefully.   Be as precise as possible in measuring the medicine. Most medicines for children are prescribed by the teaspoon. It is best to use a measuring spoon or a calibrated medicine dropper rather than a household teaspoon when measuring medicine for children. One teaspoon is equal to 5 cc or 5 ml; one-half teaspoon equals 2.5 cc or 2.5 ml. There are a variety of teaspoons and dropper-like devices available for giving liquid medicine to children. Your pharmacist can help you select one.

When giving liquid medicine hold a paper cup or small dish under the child's chin. You can retrieve the drips and put them back in your child's mouth.

Even if your baby takes a bottle, do not put medication in a bottle of juice or formula unless your doctor okays it. Some medications are rendered less effective by the acid content of juice. Or the child may not consume the whole bottle and thus will not get the whole dose of medicine.

What to do when a child spits up medicine.   Most medications are absorbed in the stomach and intestines within a half hour to forty-five minutes. If your child has retained the medicine that long it is usually unnecessary to give her another dose if she spits up. If the child spits up the medicine immediately, repeat the dosage (unless you have been advised by your doctor that a slight over-dosage may be critical, as is the case with some heart and asthma medicines). If a child spits up an antibiotic within five or ten minutes after the administration, repeat the dose.

Give the whole course of treatment.   Don't stop the medication just because your child feels better. Antibiotics often relieve symptoms within a day or two, but it takes the full course of treatment to really fight off the bacteria and keep the illness from recurring.

Make the medicine as palatable as possible.   Never tell a child that a medication is candy. This is a sure way to entice your child to explore the medicine cabinet. Do not tell a child that medication will taste good when you know it won't. Giving her a second dose will be impossible. Have a favorite food or drink close at hand to chase down the poorly tasting medicine.

Children's medicines come in liquid form, as tablets to swallow, or sometimes as chewable tablets. If your child will not take liquid medicine, crush a chewable tablet between two spoons and mix it with a small amount of applesauce, jelly, or honey. Give your child this mixture on a spoon and chase it with water or juice. You can also open up a capsule and mix the contents with applesauce or jelly. For young infants who will not take liquids and cannot chew or swallow a pill, try this: crush a chewable tablet between two spoons and add a few drops of water, making a paste of the medicine. Using your finger place a small amount of the paste on the inside of your baby's cheeks and allow her to swallow a little bit at a time.

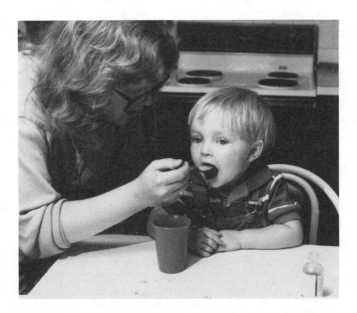

The promise of a favorite drink, ready and waiting, will help the medicine go down.

Some medications come in suppository form (acetaminophen, anti-nausea medications). These are particularly effective when a child is unable to keep down medication because of vomiting or fever. Sometimes using a suppository medication to stop vomiting is necessary before giving a child another medication orally.

Games for medicine-taking. When it comes to getting kids to take medicine, the end justifies all kinds of means. In our home, we have devised a variety of games that are only played in conjunction with taking medicine. The pleasure of the game compensates for the unpleasurable event of taking medicine. Try the run-and-bite method. Put the medicine on a spoon. Have your toddler run at you from about five feet away and stop immediately in front of the spoonful of medicine. She takes the medicine and swallows it down fast, with a juice or water chaser, and continues on her journey. Sometimes we place a favorite treat on a table just beyond the spoonful of medicine as an extra incentive.

Pill-taking in the older child. Children have great difficulty swallowing tablets. Buttering the pill or burying it in a spoonful of applesauce or jam helps it to slide down more easily. If that doesn't work try this: instead of following the natural tendency and tipping the head back to swallow a pill, have your child bend her head forward. Place the pill near the tip of her tongue. Have her take a drink of water, hold it in her mouth, and bend her head forward so that the chin touches the chest. As she swallows, she should lift her head up quickly. The pill will rise to the top of the water (toward the back of the tongue) and wash down easily with the swallow.

If the child won't take medicine for mom, use the doctor or daddy or another person as the scapegoat. My patients' parents often say, "Dr. Bill said you must take your medicine."

Stocking Your Home Medicine Cabinet

Medications

These are the most common over-the-counter and prescription medications needed for treating sick children. Depending on your child's propensity for being sick, your doctor may wish you to keep many of these on hand.

Acetaminophen	For control of fever and pain (see page 57)
Activated charcoal	For treatment of poison ingestion (see page 214).
Antacids *(Mylanta)*	For upset stomach, as directed by physician.
Antibiotic ointment *(Polysporin, Neosporin, Bactroban*)*	Antiseptic ointment for minor cuts and abrasions, as directed by physician.
Antibiotics	If you have a child who has frequent bacterial infections ask your doctor to prescribe some of the most common antibiotics in powdered form (many of the common liquid antibiotics do not store for any length of time). Have the pharmacist add directions for reconstituting the antibiotic with water. Always consult your doctor before giving antibiotics to your child.
Antihistamines *(Benadryl, Chlor-Trimeton)*	For allergic runny noses, allergies to insect bites, hay fever, or as directed by physician.
Aveeno	Soothing compound for dry itchy skin, contact dermatitis, and poison ivy.
Burn cream *(Silvadene*)*	An effective cream for promoting healing and minimizing infection; also good for lessening infection and scarring in severe chicken pox lesions or skin abrasions.

* Available by prescription only

Stocking Your Home Medicine Cabinet (continued)

Medications (continued)

Cortisone creams*	For contact dermatitis (e.g., poison ivy) and allergic reactions. Do not use unless directed by physician. Do not use on skin infections such as chicken pox. One-half percent preparations are available without prescription, one percent and above by prescription. Do not use for more than five days in succession or on the face without consulting physician.
Cough syrups	Cough syrups containing glyceryl guaiacolate or guaifenesin (expectorants) help liquify the secretions making it easier for them to be coughed up. Cough syrups containing dextromethorphan suppress the cough reflex; these are used mainly at night to help child sleep.
Decongestants (*Actifed, Novahistine, PediaCare, Rondec, Sudafed, Triaminic*)	Act by constricting the blood vessels of the nose and respiratory passages. Mainly effective in allergies; of limited use with other causes of respiratory drainage. Consult physician before use.
Diarrhea medicines	Usually not necessary in children.
Ear drops	For pain relief, *Auralgan** contains a topical anesthetic. May be used safely at night until you can talk to your doctor in the morning. Should not be used in lieu of antibiotic treatment for ear infections. *Cerumenex** and *Debrox* are solutions used to remove occlusive ear wax. For prevention of swimmer's ear, ear drops containing acidic acid are available without prescription.

* Available by prescription only

Stocking Your Home Medicine Cabinet (continued)

Medications (continued)

Eye drops or ointment	Antibiotic drops or ointment for eye infections *(erythromycin*, Tobrex*)*. Use as directed by your physician. Eye drainage in children is usually associated with ear and sinus infections which need medical attention.
Ipecac syrup	To induce vomiting of ingested poisons (see page 212). Always consult physician or poison control center before inducing vomiting.
Laxatives	As prescribed and directed by physician.
Nose drops *(Neo-Synephrine, Afrin)*	Salt-water nose drops are used in infants to loosen nasal secretions. Other types may be used in allergic runny noses. Consult physician. Nose drops often cause temporary painful burning in the child's nose.
Vomiting medications	*Emetrol,* basically a cola syrup, is available without prescription. Prescription suppositories most effective.

Other Supplies

Alcohol (rubbing)	For drying and cleansing.
Adhesive tape, 1/2" and 1" widths	For bandaging. Look for the hypoallergenic type.
Antiseptic solutions *(Hibiclens, Betadine)*	For cleansing of wounds, cuts, and abrasions.
Band-aids	As needed.
Calamine lotion	May soothe itchy skin.
Cotton balls, cotton-tip applicators	Use for cleaning orifices, applying alcohol, and other first-aid treatments.

* Available by prescription only

Stocking Your Home Medicine Cabinet (continued)

Other Supplies (continued)

Diaper rash creams	Barrier creams containing zinc oxide most effective. Severe diaper rashes are usually caused by fungus or skin irritation and may require prescription creams.
Domeboro	Soothing for itchy skin.
Elastic bandages, 2" and 4" wide	For first-aid wraps.
Enemas	Pediatric Fleet enemas. Consult physician.
Epsom salts	Soothing solution for sore muscles, itchy skin.
Gauze	4" x 4" individual squares, Kling wrap, and non-stick pads for first-aid use.
Glycerine suppositories	For relief of constipation.
Hydrogen peroxide	For removing scabs and dead tissue from a healing wound.
Measuring spoons	For giving medication.
Nasal aspirator	For removal of nasal secretions in infants.
Scissors	Blunt-end and bandage.
Steri-strips	Special band-aids used to close minor cuts.
Sunscreen	SPF 15 or higher. Products that do not contain PABA may be safer.
Tongue depressors	As needed.
Tweezers	As needed.
Thermometers	Oral and rectal.
Vaseline jelly	Useful in taking rectal temperatures and inserting suppositories.

CHAPTER 3

Common Concerns and Illnesses in the First Few Months

The first few months of a baby's life are a very special time. The baby is entirely dependent on you, and you are just getting to know him and to know yourself as a parent. Tiny babies are protected from many illnesses by the immunities they received through the placenta and by those in breast milk. But they have other health concerns that are all their own.

Common Medical Concerns in the Newborn Baby

Jaundice

Nearly all newborns develop some degree of jaundice, and parents often are anxious over what, in reality, is a variant of a normal physiological process. Jaundice is a symptom, not an illness. The yellow coloring in baby's skin and eyeballs is caused by the build-up in the blood of a yellow pigment called bilirubin. The body normally produces bilirubin when it breaks down worn-out red blood cells. This bilirubin is usually disposed of through the liver and intestines and does not reach high-enough levels in the blood to cause yellow deposits in the skin or eyes. If too many blood cells are broken up too fast, or if the liver is unable to get rid of excess bilirubin fast enough, it is deposited in the skin. Thus, the yellow color.

Jaundice in newborns may be normal (physiologic) or abnormal (pathologic). I use the term normal jaundice because almost all babies have some degree of jaundice as a normal part of their adjustment to life outside the womb. Newborns enter the world with more red blood cells than they really need. The red blood cells break down into bilirubin, and it takes a while for the newborn's immature liver and intestinal mechanisms to dispose of the excess bilirubin. Within the first few weeks, as your baby's system matures enough to dispose of the bilirubin, the jaundice subsides. As many as 90 percent of normal healthy newborns may develop physiologic jaundice, which subsides without needing treatment or causing harm.

In abnormal types of jaundice the bilirubin levels may go high enough to cause brain damage in the newborn baby. Studies have found brain damage from high levels of bilirubin only in jaundice caused by blood group incompatibilities (such as the RH factor being different in mother and baby) or in babies who were very premature or very sick. This kind of jaundice is a very different medical problem than jaundice in an otherwise healthy infant. If your baby is not extremely premature, there is no blood group incompatibility, no infection, and no disease process occurring, then jaundice is seldom a worry. Your doctor can explain to you which type of jaundice your baby has.

How to minimize jaundice in your newborn. Although normal physiologic jaundice is nothing to worry about,

I have found in my experience that much newborn jaundice is aggravated by a baby not getting enough fluids and calories in the first few days of life. Mothers who are able to room-in with their babies and breastfeed them frequently, following their cues, have babies with less jaundice and also less weight loss. One of the reasons why jaundice seems to be more common in breastfed babies is that many newborns are not fed soon enough or frequently enough, and mothers are not given proper help with breastfeeding in the hospital. As a result babies are often undernourished and slightly dehydrated, temporary factors which may not harm the baby but do contribute to jaundice. It is rarely necessary to supplement the breastfed baby with additional water or formula. Research has shown that this practice does not prevent jaundice. If supplements are necessary (because of difficulties in initiating breastfeeding), they can be given at the breast, using a nursing supplementer device.

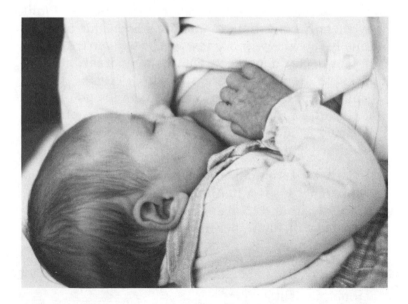

When a baby is properly positioned at the breast, his body faces his mother's and his mouth covers most of the areola.

To minimize jaundice in your newborn plan to get a
good start at breastfeeding. Be sure that your baby is
properly positioned at the breast while nursing. If you
have questions, call a La Leche League Leader or ask to
see the hospital's lactation consultant (if there is one).
Nurse frequently from birth on. This helps to bring your
milk in sooner and helps the baby get rid of bilirubin.
Have your baby room-in with you. Follow his cues and
nurse him whenever he seems hungry or in need of comfort. Breast milk helps to wash out the excess bilirubin
in the intestines. Feeding stimulates babies to have bowel
movements, and bowel movements help to get rid of
bilirubin.

Only in very rare circumstances is it necessary to stop
breastfeeding when your baby is jaundiced. There is a rare
condition called breast milk jaundice which may occur
in two to four percent of breastfed babies. This kind of
jaundice starts later than normal physiologic jaundice. It
is a poorly understood condition, but it seems that a particular substance or substances in some mothers' milk
may actually contribute to jaundice. Even this problem
normally subsides within a few weeks with no treatment,
but your doctor may recommend a temporary interrup-
tion (24 to 48 hours) in breastfeeding.

Jaundice is seldom a serious problem in and of itself.
But it causes problems when it leads to disruptions in
breastfeeding and mother-baby togetherness in the first
days after birth. Here is an all-too-common scenario:

> The baby has jaundice, and the doctors say there is no
> apparent cause for it. Although the bilirubin levels
> are only around 15 mg/dl and the baby is well, he is
> treated with phototherapy in the nursery—placed
> under a special light which decreases bilirubin
> levels—and separated from his mother. He is allowed
> to nurse only every four hours during the day and not
> much at night.

This kind of over-treatment of jaundice is usually not very
wise. When mother and baby are separated, the baby ac-

tually receives less breast milk and becomes undernourished, worsening the jaundice. The phototherapy light
also contributes to dehydration in the baby. To make up
for this the baby may be given supplemental formula or
water in bottles, and this experience with artificial nipples can confuse the baby and lead to problems nursing
at the breast. What was a normal, non-harmful physiologic process (normal jaundice) becomes a "disease"
which should never have occurred and never have been
treated. I have seen many mothers and babies who were
unable subsequently to develop a good breastfeeding relationship because of this kind of experience. Fortunately,
there are alternatives, even in situations where phototherapy is necessary. Mother and baby can both be discharged
from the hospital, and phototherapy can continue at home.
There are a number of companies around the country that
work with your doctor to provide this service. The mother-
baby separation is lessened, and the baby can breastfeed
more often in this situation. Or ask your doctor about the
use of sunlight to reduce jaundice; the naked baby can
be placed next to a closed sunny window.

Eye Discharge

Sometime during the first few weeks or months of your
baby's life, you may notice a yellow, sticky discharge from
one or both eyes. This is usually caused by a blocked tear
duct. Most infants begin tearing by three weeks of age.
These tears should drain into the nose through tiny tear
ducts at the inside corners of the eye. At birth, the nasal
ends of these ducts are sometimes covered by a thin membrane that usually breaks open shortly after birth, allowing proper drainage of tears. Often this membrane does
not fully open. The tear ducts remain plugged, and the
tears accumulate in one or both eyes. Fluid that does not
drain properly becomes infected. As a result, the discharge
from your baby's eyes may become persistently yellow,
indicating an infection in the region of the blocked tear
ducts.

Here's how to treat your baby's blocked tear ducts. Gently massage the tear duct that is located beneath the tiny "bump" in the nasal corner of each eye. Massage in an upward direction (toward the eye) about six times. Do this as often as you think of it, for example, before each diaper change. Massaging the tear duct applies pressure on the fluid trapped within the ducts and eventually pops open the membrane and clears the ducts. If you notice persistent tearing or yellow drainage from one or both eyes, your doctor will instruct you in how to massage these tear ducts and may also prescribe an antibiotic ointment to treat the infection. This problem may recur intermittently, but it usually clears by six months. Occasionally this conservative treatment does not work, and between six and nine months, it is necessary for an eye doctor to open these ducts by inserting a tiny wire into them. This is usually a short, minor office procedure. A discharge from the eyes in the first few months is almost always caused by blocked tear ducts; in the older infant and child, the problem more commonly is part of an infection in the ears and sinuses.

Thrush

Thrush is a yeast infection in a baby's mouth. It looks like cottage-cheese patches on the inner lips, tongue, and roof of the mouth. Yeast normally lives in the mouth, the intestines, and the vagina, places where there are moist mucus membranes. Because yeast thrives on milk, a baby's mouth provides an ideal environment. Many babies will have a yeast infection in the mouth in the first six months; the yeast infection may also appear in the diaper area in the form of a rash. Yeast infections are especially common following antibiotic therapy; the antibiotic kills off the good bacteria that normally keep the yeast under control. Giving acidophilus drops or powder (available from a pharmacy or health food store) while a child is on antibiotic therapy often prevents yeast infections.

Sometimes thrush can be confused with milk deposits on the tongue and mouth. The difference is that thrush cannot be easily wiped off, whereas milk can. If you attempt to scrape off a patch of thrush, the area underneath will bleed easily. Although thrush seldom bothers a baby, some babies may become irritable because of soreness in the mouth.

Thrush may be transferred to the nipples of the breast-feeding mother. Sore nipples that develop after weeks or months of comfortable nursing may indicate a thrush infection. The nipples may be tender, pink, flaky, and itchy. When a breastfed baby has thrush, it's necessary to treat the mother as well as the baby.

Treatment of Thrush

Your doctor may prescribe an antifungal medication to paint on the patches of thrush and the rest of the mucus membranes of the mouth and tongue, four times a day for ten days. Thrush often recurs, and another course of treatment is needed. Sometimes thrush can be particularly persistent, although it may not bother the baby, and a change of medication may be necessary. A persistent diaper rash may also require treatment with this oral solution even though thrush cannot be seen in the mouth.

Skin Problems

Milia

In the first few weeks, babies may have tiny, whitish, pinhead-sized bumps on the skin of the nose and sometimes on other parts of the face. These are called milia and are caused by plugging of the skin pores. They are normal and nothing to worry about. With gentle washing, these disappear within a few weeks.

Prickly Heat

Prickly heat rashes look like tiny pimples with red bases and clear centers. Prickly heat usually appears on areas of the skin where there is excessive moisture retention, such as behind the ears, between the neck folds, in the groin, or in areas where clothing fits tightly. To treat it gently wash the area in plain cool water or with a solution of baking soda (one teaspoon to a cup of water). Also, dress your baby in lightweight, loose-fitting clothing.

Cradle Cap and "Baby Acne"

Increased hormone levels at birth (perhaps similar to those in adolescence) may cause the over-production of a waxy, oily substance called sebum in the oil glands of the skin, most noticeably in the face and scalp. Plugging of these glands leads to inflammation and the formation of pimples. The medical term for this problem is seborrheic dermatitis. Unless worsened by a superimposed bacterial infection, these seborrheic rashes seldom bother a baby.

"Newborn acne" appears on the face. It is a pimply, oily rash resembling teenage acne. This will disappear eventually with gentle washing with water and a mild soap.

Cradle cap, another form of seborrheic dermatitis, is a crusty, oily, plaque-like rash on the baby's scalp, most commonly over the soft spot. A mild case of cradle cap will resemble dandruff—flaky dry skin on the scalp. It seldom needs any more treatment than gentle washing and increased humidity. Too-vigorous and too-frequent hair washing will only dry out the scalp and make the cradle cap worse.

Here's how to treat a more severe case of cradle cap. Massage vegetable oil into the crusty scales to soften them. Give the oil fifteen minutes or more to soak in, and then use a fine-tooth comb to remove the scales. Finally wash off the excess oil with shampoo. (You can skip the combing and just wash the hair if sitting still for hair-combing twice in one day is difficult for your baby.) Persistent and severe cradle cap may benefit from a mild tar shampoo. (Be careful to keep this away from baby's eyes). If cradle cap persists consult your doctor for a prescription cream.

Seborrheic dermatitis may also appear as a crusty, oily rash behind the ears and in the skin folds of the neck.

In addition to washing with warm water, a prescription cream may be needed.

Skin, especially that of a newborn baby, enjoys high humidity. This is why most of these rashes seem to be worse during the winter months when central heating dries the air. A vaporizer or humidifier in the baby's sleeping room will often lessen these rashes.

Diaper Rash

Diaper rash is a fact of civilized, bottom-covering baby life. Diapers were invented to protect the environment from baby's excrement, and baby's skin rebels at losing its freedom to enjoy the air and sunshine. A diaper held close to warm skin provides an incubator-type environment for the growth of bacteria from bowel movements. These bacteria act on chemicals in urine to produce ammonia and other skin irritants. The skin becomes inflamed and the result is diaper rash. Skin was not designed to be in prolonged contact with a wet covering. Waterproof pants covering the diaper may worsen the rash by keeping dampness in and air out.

Early on a diaper rash may resemble a red scald—a general reddening of the diaper area. With time, bacteria and/or fungi grow on this inflamed area, creating a superimposed infection in addition to the initial irritation. There may be raised pimply areas or blisters.

How to prevent and treat diaper rashes. Change wet diapers as quickly as possible. If diaper rash is a persistent problem, change your baby frequently during the night also. After each diaper change, wash the area with plain water or mild soap, rinse well, and gently blot dry. Avoid strong soaps and excessive rubbing on sensitive skin.

Allow the diaper area to "breathe." Avoid tight-fitting diapers and waterproof pants which retain moisture. Reserve the plastic pants for the times and places where a wet diaper would be a social calamity. You don't need them around home. Use rubber pads underneath your baby to protect his bedding.

"Air condition" your baby's diaper area. Expose your baby's diaper area as much as possible to the air. While he is sleeping, unfold the diaper and lay it beneath him. In warm weather, let your baby nap outside with his bare bottom exposed to the fresh air.

Diaper creams and ointments are not necessary when your baby's skin is not irritated. But at the first sign of a reddened, irritated bottom, apply a barrier cream such as zinc oxide. This helps to protect the skin from moisture and irritants. Treat the diaper rash early, before the skin breaks down and becomes infected. Barrier creams should also be used when your baby has diarrhea, such as when he is teething or has an intestinal infection, to prevent diaper rash from starting. Avoid cornstarch on the diaper area because it encourages the growth of fungi.

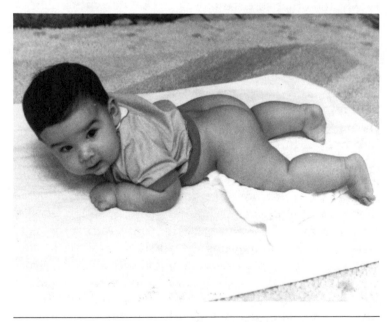

Exposure to air helps heal diaper rash.

If your baby is frequently troubled by diaper rash, experiment with both cloth diapers and disposable diapers to see which one causes fewer rashes. If you wash your own cloth diapers be sure that you use a hot wash cycle and rinse them thoroughly. Then soak the washed and rinsed diapers in a solution of one cup of vinegar to half a washing machine tub of water for one half-hour. Spin the water away, but dry the diapers without further rinsing.

Baking soda baths are particularly helpful in treating "acid-burn" types of diaper rash (a red, scald-type non-raised rash). These are particularly common after intestinal infections, which produce acidic stools, or following antibiotic treatment. Soak your baby's bottom in a baking soda solution, one tablespoon of baking soda to two quarts of water in his tub. After the soak, give a "sniff" to check for any smell of ammonia.

Yeast or fungus infections produce diaper rashes that are red, raised, rough and sore-looking, with tiny pustules. These are resistant to the above simple forms of treatment. Sometimes bacteria are also involved in these types of diaper rashes. You may need a prescription cream containing an antifungal or antibacterial agent or one containing cortisone. (Some creams contain these agents individually, some in combination.) Unless otherwise instructed by your doctor, avoid the use of cortisone creams on the diaper area for more than seven straight days.

Mothers often lament, "I do everything right. I change my baby's diapers frequently, and he still gets a rash. What have I done wrong?" Some babies have more sensitive skin than others, and no matter how hard you try they will have diaper rashes until the diapering stage is over.

Infections of the Umbilicus
It can take as as long as two weeks after birth for the umbilical cord to dry and fall off. It is normal to see a few

drops of blood when the cord falls off. Infections of the umbilical cord can be prevented with a few simple steps:

Keep the cord as dry as possible and avoid immersion baths until the cord falls off and the navel is completely dry. Do not cover the cord area with a diaper or rubber pants.

Using a cotton-tipped applicator and rubbing alcohol (or another antiseptic solution recommended by your doctor), wipe the skin around the base of the cord at least four times a day.

If the cord becomes soiled with stools, wash it off with an alcohol-soaked cotton ball and dry it well.

A slight odor from the drying cord is normal, but a particularly putrid odor may be a sign that an infection is brewing and it's time to step up the use of the antiseptic solution. If the skin around the drying cord looks normal and is not inflamed, there is seldom any reason for concern. A red, hot, swollen, and tender area the size of a half dollar around the base of the drying cord is a sign of infection.

How to Recognize
When a Tiny Infant Is Seriously Ill

The younger the baby the more subtle the signs of illness. The following symptoms indicate that a very young infant is sick:

A temperature greater than 101 °F (rectally) that lasts more than eight hours in an infant under three months.

Increasing lethargy—drowsiness, diminishing responsiveness, and an overall limp feeling. Normally tiny infants are bright-eyed, sparkly, and responsive to their environment. Their muscle tone is strong and tight.

Decreasing interest in feedings and diminished intensity of sucking lasting over eight hours.

Persistent paleness of the skin and/or blueness of the lips.

Persistent rapid breathing (greater than 60 breaths per minute during sleep, lasting for an hour or more) or labored respirations.

All of the above are serious signs that should alert parents to seek medical attention immediately. Call your doctor if your newborn shows any of these symptoms.

CHAPTER 4

Parenting the Child with Fever

Fever is the most common symptom of illness in children. An understanding of what fever really is and how to manage it is important to parenting your child when she is sick.

What Is a Fever?

A rectal temperature greater than 100.5°F (38°C) may be considered a fever. Most children have a normal body temperature of 98.6°F (37°C) orally, but normal temperature varies from 97° to 100°F (37° to 38°C). Many children show daily fluctuations in body temperature which are also normal. Your child's temperature may be lower in the morning and after resting and a degree higher during the late afternoon or during strenuous exercise.

Fever is a symptom of an underlying illness. It is not an illness itself. Your child's normal body temperature is maintained by a thermostat in a tiny part of the brain called the hypothalamus, which regulates the balance between heat produced and the heat lost by the body. Your child's temperature goes up when more heat is produced than can be released. When there is an infection in your child's body, the germs release substances called pyrogens that produce heat, thus causing a fever.

Any time there is a change from normal body temperature, your child's thermostat tries to bring the temperature back to normal. For example, when your child is cold, she shivers to produce heat. When she is warm or has a fever, the blood vessels under her skin dilate (hence her flushed cheeks) and the heart beats faster. These mechanisms cause more blood to reach the surface of the skin where it cools off, releasing excess body heat. A child with a fever also sweats so that her body cools by evaporation. She breathes faster to release warm air—the same way a dog pants to cool off during the warm summer months.

How to Take Your Child's Temperature

Take your child's temperature after she has been quiet for half an hour. A screaming baby or a child who has been running around may show a temperature one or two degrees higher than it would be after a quiet activity.

Practice "feeling" your child's temperature by placing the palm of your hand on her forehead or by kissing her forehead so that you can tell when her temperature is normal and when it is elevated. If your touch suggests that your child has a fever, confirm this by taking her temperature with a thermometer.

If your child does not seem sick at all, but the thermometer says she has a fever, shake the thermometer down well and repeat the temperature reading before panicking. If the temperature still seems high and your child still seems well, take your child's temperature with another thermometer.

Choosing a Thermometer

Buy the thermometer which is easiest for you to read. Some are easier than others. Thermometers are marked with long lines showing each degree and short lines showing each two-tenths of a degree (98.2°, 98.4°, 98.6°, etc.). To find the line of mercury that indicates temperature, hold the thermometer at the top, the end opposite from the mercury bulb. Slowly roll the thermometer between your thumb and forefinger until you notice the wide silver ribbon of mercury. You can also buy digital thermometers which simply give you a number reading.

You can take your child's temperature in three places: the rectum, the armpit (or axilla), or the mouth. Rectal temperature is one-half to one degree higher than oral temperature and axillary temperature is usually one degree lower than oral.

Shake down the thermometer with a wrist-snapping motion until the mercury column is below 95°F. Hold the thermometer tightly as you shake and do it over a bed

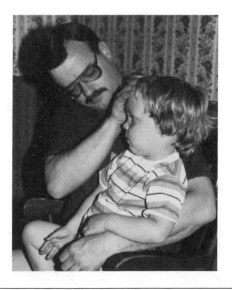

Feeling your child's forehead is the first step
to finding out if he has a fever.

or soft surface in case you drop it. Keep a temperature chart. Each time you take your child's temperature write down the time, the temperature, and the way you took the temperature (orally, rectally, or axillary). Also, next to the temperature recording, list the methods you have used to treat the fever.

How to Use a Rectal Thermometer

Using a rectal thermometer is the easiest, most accurate, and safest way to take a temperature in a child less than four years old. The only difference between rectal and oral thermometers is in the tip. The rectal thermometer is short and stubby to prevent injury to the rectum. The tip of the oral thermometer is long and thin. To take your child's rectal temperature follow these steps:

1. Shake down the thermometer. Grease the bulb end with petroleum jelly.

2. Lay your child face down across your lap.

3. Gently insert the thermometer bulb about one inch into the rectum. Allow the thermometer to seek its own path. Don't force it.

4. Hold the thermometer between your index and middle fingers with the palm of your hand and your fingers grasping your child's buttocks. This way you can hold the thermometer and keep your child from moving. Never leave a child alone with the thermometer in place.

5. Try to keep the thermometer in place for three minutes. If your child is struggling, one minute may be long enough to give a reading within a degree of the true temperature.

Using an Oral Thermometer
You can take the temperature of an older child orally. The oral thermometer has a longer, thinner shaft than the rectal thermometer and is marked "oral."

1. Shake down the thermometer as described above.

2. Have your child lie or sit quietly and place the mercury end of the thermometer under her tongue, slightly to one side. Instruct her to keep her mouth closed firmly but not to hold the thermometer with her teeth. Encourage her to breathe through her nose. Allowing the child to open her mouth to breathe may make the temperature reading inaccurate.

3. Try to keep the thermometer in place with the mouth closed for two to three minutes.

Taking an Axillary Temperature
You can use either a rectal or oral thermometer to take an axillary temperature.

1. Have your child sit on a bed, in a corner of the couch, or on your lap, and hold her firmly with one arm around her shoulder.

2. Wipe her armpit dry. Lift her arm and gently place the bulb of the thermometer into the armpit. Hold your child's arm flat against the chest, closing the armpit.

3. Allow at least three minutes to get an accurate axillary temperature.

When to Worry about Fever

It is not necessarily true that a higher fever means a sicker child. How sick your child seems generally is more important than degree of fever. Some minor illnesses can produce a very high fever, and some very serious illnesses can cause a sick child to have only a mild fever. Remember that fever is a symptom of an underlying illness, not an illness in itself. It is similar to the temperature gauge in your car which simply alerts the driver to a potential problem in the engine.

The younger the child the more worrisome a fever. Any infant under three months of age who has a temperature greater than 101 °F which persists for more than eight hours should be reported immediately to your doctor.

Two kinds of germs cause fever, viruses and bacteria. Viral infections are usually less worrisome than bacterial infections. Viral infections have these characteristics:

The fever comes on suddenly in a previously well child.

The fever is usually very high (103 ° to 105 °F).

The fever is easily brought down by the methods described below, but it may go back up again within a few hours.

The child seems sick when the fever is high but appears to feel better when the fever is brought down.

With some of the more common viruses during the first year or two parents will often remark, ''I'm surprised the fever is so high because she does not look or act that sick.'' This is especially true of the viral infection roseola which is common in the first year of life and produces a high fever (103 ° to 105 °F) for about three days; there are no other symptoms, and the child does not appear as ill as the high fever would indicate. A day or so after the fever breaks a faint generalized reddish-pink rash appears which lasts for less than twenty-four hours.

Bacterial infections usually cause a more worrisome fever pattern, characterized by the following:

The fever does not come down more than a degree or so with the usual fever-reducing methods.

The child looks and acts as sick or sicker than the degree of fever indicates.

The child does not seem to be getting any better from day to day or is getting sicker. The fever may not be changing or may be increasing.

Other signs of illness are present in addition to the fever such as: snotty nose, cough, increasing lethargy.

How to Treat Your Child's Fever

There have been recent articles in non-medical publications suggesting that parents not treat children's fevers. These are based on theories that fever mobilizes the immune system and helps the body fight off infection. There is scant experimental evidence to support this, but the question is not yet completely answered. Most physicians suggest that you treat a child's fever, mainly to make the child more comfortable and to prevent febrile convulsions. Fever can make a child miserable, causing headaches, muscle aches, and an overall unwell feeling.

I remember one day hearing a mother and grandmother arguing in my waiting room. They had brought the baby in for evaluation of fever. The grandmother was admonishing the new mother, "Wrap him up with more clothes or he'll catch cold." The mother snapped back, "He already has a cold. The heat needs to get out." Who was right? The new mother.

There are two basic ways to reduce your child's fever: give her fever-lowering medicines, such as aspirin or acetaminophen, which work by "resetting" the body's thermostat; or use cooling methods to help the body get rid of excess heat. The best way to reduce a fever is to use both methods.

You should lower your child's thermostat with medications *before* using the heat-removal procedures. When a child's body temperature is lowered using cooling methods, her thermostat reacts and produces more heat to raise the body temperature back up again. For example, removing a child's clothing and placing her in a cool bath will make her body shiver, producing heat, and her blood vessels constrict in order to conserve heat. Ultimately, this will result in a higher body temperature. But if you first give the child temperature-lowering medicines to reset the thermostat and then place her in the cool bath, her body will not react in ways that produce more heat. It is very similar to the way you might regulate heat in your home. If a room is too hot you would first lower the thermostat and then open the windows to remove the excess heat. If you open the windows without resetting the thermostat, the influx of cold air will start up the furnace and heat will continue to pour into the room.

A Step-By-Step Method to Lower Your Child's Fever
Acetaminophen is as effective as aspirin in lowering fever. (It is less effective as a pain reliever.) Acetaminophen has replaced aspirin as the fever-lowering medication of choice. It is safer and equally effective. It is not linked with Reye's syndrome as is aspirin. Reye's syndrome is a life-threatening illness that may follow a bout with influenza or chicken pox. It may be associated with the use of aspirin during these illnesses. Whether or not aspirin causes Reye's Syndrome has not been conclusively determined, but it is generally recommended that aspirin not be used routinely in children until this question is answered.

Acetaminophen is available in liquid, tablet, and suppository forms and is therefore easier to administer than aspirin tablets. You can choose the form that your child finds easiest to take. Suppositories are used in vomiting children who are unable to keep down oral medication. Although acetaminophen overdose is as serious as aspirin overdose, acetaminophen does not build up in your child's blood with prolonged use as aspirin does. Thus it is less likely to produce an overdose with routine use.

Calculating the dosage of acetaminophen. The correct dosage of acetaminophen is measured in milligrams per unit of body weight: five milligrams per pound or ten milligrams per kilogram. Acetaminophen is available in five forms:

1. Drops (used for infants under one year): 0.8 ml equals 80 milligrams acetaminophen.

2. Elixir: One teaspoon equals 5 ml equals 160 mg acetaminophen.

3. Chewable tablets: One tablet equals 80 mg acetaminophen.

4. Adult tablets: One tablet equals 325 mg acetaminophen.

5. Suppositories: One suppository equals 120 mg.

The chart will help you determine the proper dosage for your child.

Acetaminophen Dosage

Doses should be administered 4 or 5 times daily—but not to exceed 5 doses in 24 hours.

Age Group	0-3 mos	4-11 mos	12-23 mos	2-3 yrs	4-5 yrs	6-8 yrs	9-10 yrs	11-12 yrs
Weight (lbs)	6-11	12-17	18-23	24-35	36-47	48-59	60-71	72-95
Dose of acetaminophen in milligrams (mg)	40	80	120	160	240	320	400	480
Drops (80 mg/0.8 ml) dropperfuls	½	1	1½	2	3	4	5	—
Elixir (160 mg/5 ml) tsp.	—	½	¾	1	1½	2	2½	3
Chewable tablets (80 mg each)	—	—	1½	2	3	4	5	6
Suppositories (120 mg each)	One suppository/year of age 4 times/day							

Other ways to lower your child's fever. After giving your child acetaminophen to reset her thermostat and lessen heat production, use the following methods to help remove the excess heat from her system.

Undress your child completely, or at most, dress her in light, loose-fitting clothing. This allows excess heat to escape her body into the cooler air. Well-meaning friends may advise you to bundle your child up when she has a fever, but this will only cause the body to retain heat. I have seen infants with fevers come into my office bundled up like Eskimos or little burritos—in southern California. This only raises the child's temperature.

Keep your child's environment cool. Decrease the temperature inside by opening a window slightly or using an air conditioner or fan. A draft will not bother the child. Cool air helps remove the heat that is radiating from her body. It is all right for a child to go outside when she has a fever. The fresh air is good for her.

Give your child a lot of **extra fluids.** Fever causes your child to lose body fluids. Give her cool, clear liquids in small amounts frequently throughout the day. Nutritious popsicles are a favorite source of fluids for sick children.

Ways to Control a Fever

---

1. Appropriate doses of acetaminophen every four hours.

2. Dress or cover your child very lightly.

3. Encourage your child to drink plenty of fluids.

4. Keep the environment cool.

5. If the fever does not go below 103 °F (39 °C) with the above steps, place your child in a tepid bath or shower.

6. If the fever comes down two degrees and your child looks and acts better, do not worry. If the fever does not come down and your child continues to get sicker, call your doctor.

7. Do not awaken a feverish sleeping child. The rest is more important than treating the fever.

Place your child in a **cooling bath**. If, in spite of trying all the above fever-lowering measures, your child's
fever remains above 103 °F (39.5 °C), or if she continues
to be uncomfortable with the fever, try using a bath to
bring the fever down. Place your child in a tub of water
and run the water all the way up to her neck. The water
temperature should be warm enough not to be uncomfortable but cooler than body temperature. If a young child
protests and begins to cry, try sitting in the bathtub with
her and amusing her with her favorite floating toys. Crying and struggling will only increase a temperature. If your
child dislikes the bath, try standing with her in a shower.
Keep your child in the cooling bath or shower for twenty
to thirty minutes. This should bring down the temperature a couple of degrees. During the bath, rub her with
a wash cloth to stimulate circulation to the skin and increase heat loss. After the bath, gently pat your child dry,
leaving a little bit of dampness on her skin which will

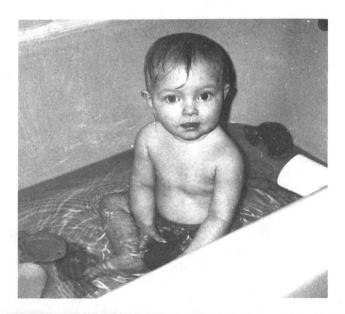

A bath will bring a fever down a couple of degrees.

evaporate and produce a further cooling effect. Do not use alcohol rubs to bring down a fever, because the vapors are toxic and they produce shivering. If your child's temperature zooms back up again, repeat the tub bath.

When to Call Your Doctor about Fever
Unless your child seems very sick, try the above fever-lowering techniques before calling your doctor. Your doctor is interested in how sick your child looks and acts rather than how high the temperature went. When you do call, one of the first questions your doctor will ask you is how your child has responded to temperature-lowering methods.

Here are some general guidelines on when to call your doctor about a child's fever:

Any fever in an infant less than three months of age which persists more than eight hours should be immediately reported to your doctor.

Any fever that cannot be lowered by using the above methods should be reported to your doctor, especially if the child is rapidly becoming more ill.

If obvious signs and symptoms, such as ear pain, severe cough, sore throat, or pain with urination, are associated with a fever, call your doctor since these could indicate a bacterial infection.

If the child is becoming increasingly drowsy, pale, and lethargic, and does not respond to the above fever-lowering mechanisms, call your doctor, regardless of the degree of fever.

Fever in an otherwise well child who has no obvious signs of pain and no other symptoms usually can wait for a day or so before you call the doctor.

How to report your child's fever to your doctor.   When you talk to your doctor by phone or bring the child to the office, have the following information ready:

1. How the fever began. Did it come on suddenly in a previously well child and shoot up very fast or did it begin very gradually and increase slightly each day as your child became sicker?

2. What does the fever chart look like? What have you done to control the fever and how has your child responded?

3. What other symptoms does your child have (earache, sore throat, vomiting, diarrhea, etc.)?

4. Does your child seem to be getting sicker, less sick, or staying the same?

5. How worried are you?

Can Fever Be Dangerous?

In most children, the fever itself is not dangerous. It does make children very uncomfortable, creating a general feeling of achiness. The main reason for trying to control high temperatures in young children is to avoid febrile convulsions. The young child's brain does not tolerate sudden temperature fluctuations and may react to them with a convulsion. It is not so much how high the temperature is, but rather, how fast it rises that causes convulsions. The younger the child the more susceptible she is to a convulsion caused by fever. Febrile convulsions are unusual in children over the age of five. All of the previously described measures for controlling your child's temperature can help to prevent febrile convulsions.

What to do if your child has a febrile convulsion.   Most febrile convulsions last only a few seconds. They are very alarming to parents but do not harm the child. Your child may shake all over, and her eyes may roll back; she may turn very pale, drool, and arch her back and stiffen out her limbs. It may seem like an eternity, but convulsions usually last no longer than ten to twenty seconds. Only a convulsion which causes the child to stop breathing for a couple of minutes is likely to do any harm. If a convulsion begins, undress your child immediately and take her into a cool shower. The convulsions will stop as soon as the fever goes down. It is common and normal for a child to fall into a deep sleep for an hour or so following a febrile convulsion.

CHAPTER 5

Respiratory Illnesses

Runny noses are the hallmark of small children in wintertime. Respiratory illnesses range from simple sniffles to pneumonia. Care and attention in the early stages can often prevent more serious problems from developing.

Colds

What is a cold? In medical terms, colds are called upper respiratory infections. Germs, either viruses or bacteria, infect the lining of the air passages in the nose, sinuses, throat, ears, and larynx. The lining reacts by swelling and secreting mucus; this produces the many symptoms associated with colds. The runny nose and postnasal drip are caused by the accumulation of mucus. Sneezes and coughs are the body's way of trying to clear this mucus. Swelling of the lining of the nose causes a child to breathe noisily through the mouth. Swelling of the veins and tissues beneath the eyelids causes a bluish discoloration which contributes to the peaked look of a child with a cold. Swelling of the tonsils and adenoids together with mucus secretions account for the throaty noises that children usually have with a cold. These secretions drip down the throat when the child lies on his back; this accounts for coughs and noisy breathing being worse at night. Swelling of the larynx and vocal cords causes a croupy, seal-bark cough.

The phrase "to catch a cold" is medically accurate, although it may be more accurate to say that the cold catches you. Colds are caused by coming in contact with germs. Colds are not caused by standing in drafts, by going without a hat, by getting wet feet, by not dressing warmly enough, or by not eating vegetables. Colds are caught when cold germs are transmitted from one person to another.

These germs usually travel through the air by a mechanism called droplet transmission. In other words, the germs reside in the tiny particles that are released into the air when someone coughs or sneezes. (That's why your child should cover his nose and mouth when he coughs or sneezes.) When cold germs enter your child's respiratory passages, they set up camp for a while before symptoms begin. This is called the incubation period, the time between exposure to a germ and the onset of symptoms. Most cold germs have a seven-to-fourteen-day incubation period, some as short as four days. So if your child visited a friend with a cold yesterday and comes down with symptoms today, you shouldn't blame that friend. He probably picked up this cold germ from someone else seven to fourteen days ago.

Most children will get around six colds per year during the first few years. As the child grows, his immunity to various germs increases, and the number and severity of colds gradually decrease. Most colds do occur in the winter months, from November to February, although the cold weather is not to blame. Children are in closer contact during the winter, the air is dryer and circulates less in centrally heated houses, and it may be that cold germs like to come indoors during the winter.

Colds in Babies

In the early months, what looks like a cold may not really be one. It may be only a case of "infant sniffles." In the first few months babies breathe primarily through the nose. Their nasal passages are easily clogged with lint from blankets and clothing, dust, even milk residue. Because these nasal passages are small, even a slight amount of clogging can cause noisy, uncomfortable breathing.

How to clean your baby's nose. Treat the sniffles with a good "nose blow." Of course your baby is too young to blow his own nose. Instead, you have to clean it out. Prepare some salt-water nose drops—about a quarter teaspoon of salt to eight ounces of water. You can also buy saline (salt-water) nose drops at the drug store. Using a plastic dropper gently squirt a few drops in each nostril. The salt water loosens the nasal secretions, especially in the morning when they may be thick and dried. The nose drops also stimulate your baby to sneeze or cough. Gently suck out the loosened nasal secretions using a nasal aspirator, a rubber bulb syringe which is available at any drug store.

To ease or help prevent the sniffles, put a humidifier or vaporizer in your baby's room during the winter months. This counteracts the drying effect of central heating on the nasal passages. Remove common dust collectors such as stuffed animals, feather pillows, and fuzzy blankets from your baby's sleeping environment. Some babies are allergic to dust. Keep your baby away from cigarette smoke which can irritate his breathing passages.

"Two-month colds." Around the second month, your baby may have a gurgling cough, and you may feel a rattle in his chest. He seems generally well and happy, with no runny nose—he is just noisy. Medically speaking, this "two-month cold" is not really a cold since it is not caused

by infection. Around two to three months of age babies begin to produce a lot of saliva, often more than they can swallow comfortably. Some of this saliva stays in the back of the throat. Air passing through it produces gurgly noises. When you place your hand on the baby's back or chest, the rattle you hear and feel is not really coming from the chest but from the vibrations produced by air passing through saliva in the back of the throat.

Saliva noises usually lessen when babies fall asleep, because saliva production slows down during sleep. Placing your baby on his stomach to sleep will allow the saliva to drool out or pool in the cheeks instead of the throat. Your baby will not choke on these secretions and will eventually learn to swallow excess saliva. No medicines are necessary. During the pre-teething stage from four to six months, there is another surge in saliva production which may again cause gurgly throat sounds and an occasional hacking cough. By six months, when your baby is sitting up most of the time and the teeth begin to appear, the swallowing mechanism matures and these throat sounds gradually disappear.

Treating the Common Cold

In the usual cold caused by a virus, a child is noisy and sneezy but does not act very sick. The nasal discharge is clear and watery—a runny nose. Your child's temperature is normal or only slightly elevated, and each day the cold seems to bother the child less, usually subsiding toward the end of one week. Your child may have a diminished appetite, wakefulness, tiredness during play, headaches, muscle aches, and a generally unwell appearance.

There are several things you can do to lessen the discomfort of your child's cold and to prevent it from becoming worse. Rest, extra fluids, and acetaminophen for fever are important in the treatment of a cold. It's also helpful to do what you can to keep the mucus discharge thin and moving.

Just as still water in a pond stagnates and becomes a breeding ground for all kinds of organisms, so do mucus secretions in children. Secretions trapped in the sinuses, Eustachian tubes (the passages between the middle ear and the back of the throat), and ears provide an attractive medium for bacteria to multiply and eventually cause a bacterial infection.

Drinking plenty of fluids and using a cool mist vaporizer help thin the secretions and allow your child to get rid of them more easily by coughing and sneezing. The child under two, or even under three, has great difficulty blowing his nose. You may have to clean out his nose as you would an infant's, using a nasal aspirator (see page 65). You can teach a young child to blow his nose by helping him pretend that he is blowing out a candle using only the air from his nose; remind him to keep his mouth closed. Encourage the older child to blow out, not sniff in. When children cough up secretions they usually swallow them. This is why children who cough a lot during a cold may also vomit.

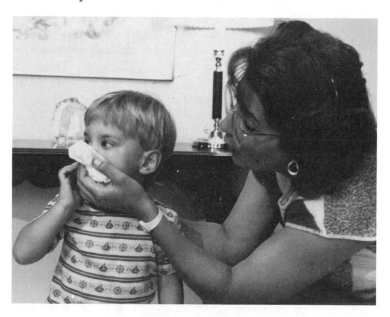

Teach and encourage your child to blow his nose when he has a cold.

Medications for colds.   The common cold is caused by
a virus, and therefore antibiotics are usually unnecessary.
Antibiotics are effective against bacteria, but not against
viruses.

Over-the-counter remedies for colds are formulated
to relieve cold symptoms. There are four basic kinds of
over-the-counter remedies: decongestants, which dry up
the secretions; expectorants, which thin the secretions and
make them easier to cough up; cough suppressants, which
suppress the cough reflex, and nose drops, which act lo-
cally to dry up nasal secretions.

Over-the-counter remedies should be used wisely in
dealing with the symptoms of a cold. **Decongestants,**
which dry up secretions and shrink the swelling of the
lining of the respiratory passages, may actually make the
secretions thicker and more difficult to cough up. Also,
some research suggests that decongestants may interfere
with the normal clearing of respiratory passages. The lining of the respiratory passages contains tiny hairs called
cilia, which push the secretions along, allowing the child
to cough them up more easily. Decongestants may interfere with the action of the cilia and allow secretions to
stagnate, making them more difficult to remove and more
susceptible to bacterial infection. If the child's cold seems
to be primarily in his chest, decongestants may only
worsen the situation.

In my experience decongestants are most effective in
controlling secretions caused by allergy: runny nose, watery eyes, and postnasal drip. If your child is not particularly bothered by the secretions (he is sleeping well and
breathing normally), I would advise against the use of
decongestants. If the nose is constantly stuffed up and the
postnasal drip is very annoying and even wakes the child
at night, decongestants may be helpful. Decongestants often have undesirable side effects, including drowsiness,
excitability, night-waking, and rapid heart beat. Some parents have told me that their child gets "squirrelly" or
"hyper" on decongestants.

I have noticed a wide range of effects among children. Some experience few side effects, some no side effects (or beneficial effects); some children cannot tolerate decongestants at all.

Expectorants are designed to loosen the secretions in the lower breathing passages leading to the lungs, enabling your child to cough up secretions. They are used primarily for lower airway congestion or to "loosen the cough." They are not effective in drying up a runny nose.

Cough suppressants act by suppressing the cough reflex. Remember, coughing up the secretions is a normal body defense, and secretions that stagnate in the lower airway may become infected with bacteria. Unless directed by your doctor, cough suppressants should be used only at night, to help the child sleep. A coughing child should be allowed to go ahead and cough during the day. The most effective over-the-counter remedies for cough usually contain a combination of an expectorant and a cough suppressant.

Nose drops may help a persistently runny nose that is really bothering a child. Bear in mind that nose drops must be used with great caution in children. While nose drops bring immediate relief to a stuffy nose, allowing the child to breathe more easily, the frequent use of nose drops may actually worsen nasal congestion. Nose drops shrink the mucus-producing vessels and lining of the nose. As their effect wears off, there may be a rebound effect that produces more congestion than before.

Limit the use of nose drops to no more than three times a day for no longer than three straight days. Check with your doctor for advice on the best nose drops to use, depending on your child's age.

When Is a Cold More Than a Cold?
The common cold is usually caused by a virus and subsides within a week or so. However, it is important for parents to recognize when a cold is becoming more than a cold and needs medical treatment. The following guide-

lines will help you decide when to take your child to a doctor for treatment of a cold.

Determine how much the cold is bothering your child. If your child is happy and playful, eats well, sleeps well, and is not particularly bothered by the cold, then it most likely is a viral infection. The cold is simply a nuisance and probably will subside with the simple suggestions listed above. If, however, the cold is increasingly bothering your child, interfering with his sleep, play, appetite, and general well-being, and it doesn't seem to be going away, it is wise to seek medical attention.

Check the mucus coming from your child's nose. If the secretions are clear and watery and your child is generally happy, the cold is most likely caused by a virus. If the discharge from the nose is becoming yellowish-green and thick and stays that way throughout the day, he probably has a bacterial infection, especially if he is becoming increasingly cranky and is awakening more at night. Nasal discharge usually appears yellow in the morning, after awakening, because of accumulations during the night. If the nasal secretions become clear during the day and your baby is happy, he probably has nothing more than a common cold.

The eyes are often a mirror of a cold's severity. Glassy, reddened eyes are often a clue that a child is ill. If your child has a persistent yellow drainage from his eyes, he very likely has an underlying sinus or ear infection and should be examined by your doctor. In my office we strongly suggest that every child with a cold who has yellow drainage from the eyes come in for an examination. I have found that at least 50 percent of children with a combination of a cold and yellow drainage in the eyes will have an underlying ear and/or sinus infection—more than just a common cold.

Antibiotics for Colds?

Viral infections generally do not need antibiotics, but bacterial infections do. When your doctor examines a child with a cold, he or she is trying to judge whether the infection is caused by a virus or by bacteria. Your doctor looks into your child's nose, throat, and ears and listens to his chest in order to determine whether there are any signs of bacterial infection. Usually bacterial infections will cause sore-looking ears, thick, "snotty" drainage in the nose and throat, an inflamed throat, swollen glands under the jaws, and noises in the chest. If none of these signs appear, your doctor may say to you, "This is a viral infection which does not need an antibiotic. Your child should get better by simply giving him plenty of fluids and cleaning out his nose. But call me if he gets worse."

Keep in mind that you are going to your doctor for consultation and advice, not necessarily for medication. Do not be disappointed if your doctor doesn't prescribe anything. It often requires more discretion *not* to treat an illness with antibiotics. Viral infections do not usually need antibiotics. The use of an antibiotic may lead to yeast infections and the development of resistance to that antibiotic, making it ineffective when used at a later date; therefore, antibiotics should not be used unless necessary. Do call your doctor if your child gets worse, since viral infections may progress to bacterial infections and a change of treatment may be necessary. Most doctors have encountered situations where they see a child for evaluation of a cold a week or two after the child was seen by another doctor. The parents may feel that the first doctor did not treat the cold properly, because now the child is getting sicker and the second doctor has prescribed an antibiotic. It is probable that when the first doctor saw the

---

When to Take a Child with a Cold to the Doctor

Dr. Bill's Rule

Happy child + clear nasal drainage = no need for medical attention

Increasingly unhappy child + increasingly snotty nose = time to visit the doctor

ALWAYS check with your doctor if your child's cold is getting worse.

child the problem *was* simply a cold which should have gone away by itself, but didn't. Common colds in children sometimes progress into ear, sinus, and chest infections, and thus need antibiotics. Always check back with your doctor if your child's cold gets worse.

When Is a Cold Contagious?

A cold is most contagious in the very early stages, even before you notice cold symptoms. Usually, the longer the cold persists, the less contagious it is. As a general guide, the sicker the child, the more important it is to keep him away from other children. If a child has a clear runny nose and no fever and is not acting sick (he's just noisy, due to sniffles and coughing), it is usually unnecessary to quarantine him from other children. If, however, the child is coughing profusely, has a snotty nose and yellow drainage from the eyes, is running a fever, and is generally ill, consider him contagious and keep him away from other people's children for a few days. Colds are spread from droplet infection (through the air on the tiny particles coughed or sneezed from your child's respiratory tract), so it takes close contact to transmit a cold. I do not really believe that colds are easily transmitted by children handling each other's toys, but colds can be transmitted by germs on the hands. Encourage your child to keep his hands away from his nose and mouth. Frequent handwashing can help prevent the spread of colds.

How to Communicate with Your Doctor about Your Child's Cold

Before phoning your doctor have the following information available:

Name and age of child

When the cold began

How the cold has progressed—whether it is getting better, worse, or staying the same

How much the cold is bothering your child's sleep, play, appetite

The nature of the drainage: clear and runny or thick, yellowish green, and snotty

The primary symptoms: fever, nasal discharge, eye drainage, cough, earache, etc.

Symptoms that have appeared only recently, as the cold has progressed: lethargy, paleness, pain in ears, around nose, in the throat

Other symptoms: swollen glands, rash, persistent vomiting, drowsiness, difficulty walking, etc.

How worried you are.

The Persistent Cough

Some coughs hang on a long time. They can linger for several weeks, even though a child does not seem sick. The cough is not too bad during the day, but the child coughs a lot at night. A lingering cough can become a real nuisance, both to the child and to the whole family.

A lingering cough is usually caused by a lingering virus which produces a type of viral bronchitis that may take four to six weeks to subside completely. If your child seems almost completely well during the day, is able to

---

How to Treat a Cold

---

1. Rest and get plenty of extra fluids.
2. Clean out the nose. Blow nasal secretions out, don't sniff them in.
3. Increase humidity in the environment.
4. Avoid contact with respiratory irritants such as cigarette smoke.
5. If the cold is getting worse, contact your doctor for advice on over-the-counter medication or an office visit.

play normally and attend school, has a good appetite, no fever and no symptoms except for the cough, this is usually nothing more than a lingering virus which will go away eventually. As with most respiratory infections, treatment consists of keeping the mucus thin and moving, encouraging the child to drink lots of fluids, and using an expectorant during the day and a cough suppressant at night. Periodically clap on your child's chest using the chest physiotherapy technique outlined on pages 101-102. Use a vaporizer in the child's sleeping environment. Clean the vaporizer regularly.

Any cough that persists longer than a few weeks, especially if it is getting worse or is accompanied by other signs of illness, should be checked by your doctor. It may be a sign of chronic sinus infection or the presence of a foreign body in the lungs. Sometimes a child with a lingering cough may go several days without seeming sick, but then suddenly begins to run a fever and become more ill as the cough worsens. This usually means that the child has retained a plug of mucus in the airway which has become infected and needs treatment. In children, it is common for a secondary bacterial infection to begin while a viral infection is healing.

Persistent Cough in an Infant
A group of viruses called whooping cough-like viruses may be responsible for coughing bouts in infants under a year of age. The baby may seem completely well except for a slight runny nose, but then suddenly he goes into a coughing spasm. He produces ten to twenty rapid staccato coughs and becomes very red in the face. He may spit up or even vomit. At the end of the approximately ten-second coughing spasm, the infant takes a prolonged deep breath which may produce a whooping type of sound. The baby is often reasonably well for another few hours, and then the coughing spasm begins again.

This infection is usually caused either by whooping cough or another virus, either one of which causes an inflammation of the lower airways. The inflammation causes the airways to secrete mucus, and your baby coughs to gradually move the secretions up into the throat where he can swallow them. Watching this cough, you will get the impression that the baby is trying to move the problem up through his bronchi and that all is well after he has dislodged the obstruction.

It is very important to use measures to calm your child and humidify his environment. (See the section on treating croup, page 96.) You should seek medical attention for this type of cough. Your doctor may suggest hospitalizing the baby for a few days to be sure that the mucus is not obstructive or he or she may instruct you on home treatment. These lingering coughs in infants are usually caused by viruses and may take several weeks to subside. Treatment consists of keeping the mucus thin and moving and preventing a bacterial infection from developing.

Coughs in Children

When Not to Worry

The child has no fever and appears generally well.

The child coughs during the day but sleeps well at night.

The cough does not interfere with eating, playing, school, or sleep.

The cough begins gradually, gets worse for a day or two, and then begins to improve.

When to Seek Medical Attention

The cough begins suddenly and is relentless. The child may have gotten something harmful (a peanut, a part of a toy) into his lungs.

The cough grows progressively worse.

The cough wakes the child at night.

The cough is accompanied by fever, chills, and other symptoms of general illness.

The child is coughing up thick yellow sputum.

The cough is accompanied by severe allergies.

Ear Infections

Ear infections are a common reason for seeking medical help during the first few years. The medical term for them is **otitis media**, which means inflammation of the middle ear. Parents should have an understanding of the causes, prevention, and treatment of ear infections.

Why Children Get Ear Infections So Frequently

An understanding of the anatomy and function of the middle ear helps to explain why ear infections are such a common childhood problem. Children harbor germs in the secretions of the nose and throat. Because the Eustachian tube connects the middle ear with the back of the mouth and throat, it is easy for germs to travel into the ear during a cold. The Eustachian tube often does not function adequately in children. It has two main functions: one, to allow air to enter the middle ear from the throat, thereby equalizing pressure on both sides of the eardrum allowing it to vibrate freely, and two, to drain the middle ear of fluid which may collect during a cold. A child's Eustachian tube is short, wide, and straight and is set at a horizontal angle; all of these characteristics allow secretions and germs to travel more easily from the throat up into the middle ear. As your child grows, the Eustachian tube becomes longer and narrower and slants at a more acute angle; this makes it more difficult for germs and fluid to collect in the middle ear.

During a cold, fluid accumulates in the middle ear. Fluid trapped anywhere in the body will usually get infected. The ear is one of the most common places for fluid to get trapped in young children because the Eustachian tube does not yet function properly. The fluid trapped in the middle-ear cavity acts like a culture medium for germs to grow. The infected fluid accumulates behind the eardrum, pressing on it and producing intense pain. If the pressure from the trapped fluid builds up too much, it can rupture the eardrum, and you may notice the fluid draining outside the ear canal. Your child's hearing depends upon the eardrum and the structures in the middle ear vibrating properly. Repeated infections cause scars on the eardrum which prevent it from vibrating properly and thus interfere with hearing. For this reason it is very important to be vigilant about proper medical treatment of your child's ear infections, especially during the early years when your child's speech and language abilities are developing. If your child's hearing is lost periodically during these formative years, he may show some speech delay and have language problems that can affect his school performance years later. Behavior problems may also accompany chronic ear infections.

Preventing Ear Infections
Because of the structure of the Eustachian tubes, many children have one or two ear infections each year. The following suggestions may help lessen the frequency and severity of these infections:

1. Breastfeed your infant for as long as possible. Breastfed infants have fewer ear infections.

2. Control allergies. Allergic symptoms often cause fluid to build up in the middle ear. Inhalant allergies (cigarette smoke, dust) and food allergies (especially to dairy products) may contribute to ear infections.

3. Treat colds early and appropriately. If your child has a history of ear infections associated with colds, it may be wise to seek medical attention early in the cold's development, before it settles in your child's ears.

4. If your baby is bottle-fed, feed him in an upright position. This lessens the chances of milk or formula entering the Eustachian tube from the throat, causing inflammation which may lead to a middle-ear infection. (Breastfeeding lying down seldom causes ear infections because the swallowing mechanism is different and breast milk is less

irritating to tissues. However, if a breastfeeding infant has recurring ear infections, it might be helpful to avoid breastfeeding while lying down until the child is older.)

How to Recognize an Ear Infection

The older child can tell you when his ear hurts, but it is often difficult for a parent to recognize an ear infection in a child who does not yet talk. If your baby has a cold, is cranky and irritable, and has nasal drainage that has become thick and yellowish-green, it is possible that he has an ear infection. Consult your doctor. Teething symptoms are sometimes confused with ear infections, but when teething your baby should look generally well and his throat and nose secretions should not be persistently yellow or green. Yellow drainage from the eyes accompanying a cold is another possible sign of an underlying ear infection. A breastfed baby may be reluctant to nurse on one side if his ear is bothering him, or he may show a change in his sucking pattern.

Ear infections often bother a child more at night. When he is lying down on his side, the fluid trapped in the middle ear presses directly down on the eardrum. You may notice that your baby seems to feel better when you hold him in an upright position or when he stands up in the crib. This is because there is less pressure on the eardrum

---

Symptoms of Ear Infections

Persistent worsening cold

Increasingly thick and yellow secretions from nose and/or eyes

Crankiness, irritability, poor appetite

Frequent night-waking

Unwillingness to lie down

Drainage from ear

Fever (may or may not be present)

Pain in the ear

when the fluid pools in the bottom of the middle ear, rather than directly against the eardrum. This explains how a child can be up all night with ear pain but feel better the next day. You should still take him to the doctor that day, even though he feels better; this will prevent the same problem from occurring the next night and interrupting your sleep, your child's, and your doctor's.

In the absence of other signs and symptoms, pulling at the ear is not a reliable sign of ear infection. Some infants will pull at their ear during teething since teething pain may travel up the jaw bone into the area of the ear. Also, some babies just like to pull at their ears.

Ruptured eardrums. It is important for parents to be vigilant about recognizing the signs of ruptured eardrums. If the pressure from fluid trapped in the middle ear builds up too much, the eardrum may rupture and the fluid will drain out of the ear canal. This fluid resembles the secretions from a runny nose. You may notice it on your child's pillow in the morning and think that it has come from the nose. However, if you look at your child's ear carefully you will notice the fluid collecting around the opening to the ear. Or there may be dried, crusted secretions at the entrance to the ear canal. Once the ear drum ruptures and the pressure is released, the child feels better. But this is a false improvement. The infection still needs to be treated to allow the perforated area of the eardrum to heal. Frequent rupture of the eardrum and the consequent scarring can result in permanent hearing loss.

Fluid in the middle ear. Your doctor may tell you that your child has fluid in the middle ear—even during a routine well-baby exam. This is the fluid that accumulates during an allergic reaction or cold. Sometimes the fluid that builds up in the middle ear does not become infected and may not produce significant pain. This is called **serous otitis media** (serous means fluid). The fluid presses on the eardrum and restricts its movement, thus diminishing your child's hearing. Even if there is no infection, most children show some signs of diminished hearing. Be on the lookout for this and other changes in behavior during colds or bouts with allergies; some children may show balance problems as a result of fluid in the middle ear. This may be the only way that you will know that your child has fluid in his middle ear. Sometimes this fluid may drain out by itself, but more often it goes on to become infected, necessitating medical treatment.

Treating Ear Infections

After your doctor diagnoses an ear infection, he or she will usually prescribe an antibiotic. The strength of the antibiotic and the duration that it is to be taken will depend on the severity of the infection and your child's past history of response to treatment.

The healing process for ear infections usually has two phases. Your child should feel better within one or two days after starting the medication, and he may seem perfectly well within two or three days. This is the first phase. During this time most of the germs have been killed by the antibiotic and the pressure of the fluid is lessened so that your child's pain is nearly gone. The second phase involves the gradual absorption or drainage of this fluid from the middle ear through the Eustachian tube. For this reason, it is important to complete the prescribed duration of treatment. If you stop giving the antibiotics just because your child feels better, the fluid that remains in the middle ear may become reinfected, and the whole treatment process must start all over again. Most ear infections require at least seven to ten days of antibiotic treatment.

Follow-up ear exams.   It is also extremely important for your doctor to recheck your child's ear as soon as the prescribed antibiotic is finished. Your doctor may decide to give your child a milder antibiotic for a while longer if the infection is not cleared completely. Partially treated ear infections are a common cause of permanent hearing deficits; therefore, follow-up checks with your doctor are extremely important.

I cannot overemphasize the importance of keeping your follow-up appointments with your doctor. I have seen many children who failed their hearing test on school entry. When you review the history of these children you discover that they had frequent ear infections which were not treated long enough, or the child's ears were not rechecked following treatment— because she seemed "all better." Even though the child seems perfectly well, fluid may remain in the middle ear for a long time, gradually becoming thicker—what physicians call "glue ear." It may require surgical drainage in order to restore the ear to normal hearing. While it may seem expensive to pay for two or three (or even more) office visits to be certain the ear infection is completely gone, an ear infection that is not completely eradicated usually creates more medical expense in the long run.

Self-Help for Middle-of-the-Night
(and Middle-of-the-Day) Earaches
Should you call your doctor in the middle of the night if your child awakens with an earache? Pediatricians, like parents, have given up the right to a full night's sleep, but it is seldom necessary to consult your doctor in the middle of the night if your child awakens with an earache, unless he seems seriously ill all over. The only treatment your doctor can prescribe for a middle-of-the-night ear infection is an antibiotic. Since antibiotics may take as long as twelve hours to have any effect, they will not immediately relieve the pain, and anyway, you may have difficulty finding a drug store open in the wee hours of the morning. Try the following pain-relieving measures instead. These will help to relieve pain in a daytime earache as well, until the antibiotics begin to take effect.

Give your child acetaminophen to help relieve the pain. (See page 57 for dosage.) It is appropriate and safe to double the first dose.

Warm some cooking oil, such as olive oil or vegetable oil, and squirt a few drops into the sore ear. Massage the outer edge of the ear canal to move the drops down toward the eardrum to relieve the pain.

Place a warm heating pad or hot water bottle against the ear. (But don't leave the heating pad in place while the child is sleeping.)

Encourage your child to lie with the sore ear up or sit your child upright, and try to help him go back to sleep in that position.

Repeat the pain reliever and the oil regimen again in three hours, if your child awakens. Ask your doctor about analgesic ear drops that you can keep in your home pharmacy for these middle-of-the-night earaches. These pain-relieving measures will often tide your child over until morning when you can consult your doctor. Even though your child may feel better in the morning, it is still wise to call the doctor.

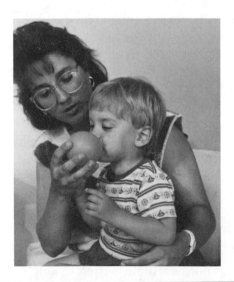

Trying to blow up a balloon creates air pressure that opens the Eustachian tubes and relieves earache pain.

Eustachian tube exercises.   Have you ever experienced
ear pain in an airplane upon take-off or landing? You may
have tried all kinds of facial contortions, yawning, swallowing, and chewing gum in order to make your ears
"pop" and relieve the pressure. The pop was your Eustachian tubes opening.

Opening the Eustachian tubes can also relieve earache
pain and facilitate drainage of middle-ear fluid in children.
The school-age child can be taught to pop his ears by blowing his nose *gently* (sudden vigorous blowing can actually
worsen Eustachian tube congestion), swallowing, chewing gum, or holding his nose while trying to blow air out
through it. The preschool child usually cannot do these
things. I have found that blowing up balloons is an effective "ear popper" for preschool children. First, stretch the
balloon to make it easier for your child to blow it up. Then,
encourage your child to blow. Even though he may not
succeed in fully inflating the balloon, creating the air pressure needed to make the balloon expand may open the
Eustachian tubes and relieve ear pain. (Young children
should always be supervised when playing with uninflated
balloons. They can cause choking.) Party favors—the ones
you blow into to unroll a long tongue-like projection—
also help to open the Eustachian tubes. Blowing against
some resistance is necessary to inflate the Eustachian
tubes; blowing soap bubbles won't do the trick.

Recurrent Ear Infections

Some children have one ear infection after another during the first few years. Parents are usually frustrated by
the recurrence of these infections and the continued medical expenses. Although children are usually very resil-
ient when it comes to illness, children with recurrent ear
infections often begin to show signs of deteriorating behavior, such as chronic irritability. I call this an "ear personality." This is common in children with recurrent ear
infections simply because they do not feel well or hear
well. One of the main changes parents notice after recurrent ear infections are finally brought under control is that

their child behaves better. Remember, a child who feels right usually acts right.

There are ways to prevent recurrent ear infections. The usual reason for recurrent ear infections is that the previous infection has never completely cleared up. A child is given antibiotics for a specified length of time and seems better, but a pool of fluid remains stuck behind the eardrum. This fluid acts as a growth medium for bacteria, and a week or two later the child is back in the doctor's office with another ear infection. If your child's ear infections are occurring frequently and lasting a long time, your doctor may suggest a prevention regimen aimed at preventing the fluid from reaccumulating in the middle ear and preventing the fluid which does accumulate from becoming infected. What follows is the regimen we have used successfully in my office for the last ten years.

Strict allergy control. Do some detective work to determine what possible allergens your child may be exposed to. The most common are dairy products, cigarette smoke, animal dander, and dust from dust-collecting stuffed animals. These allergens should be removed from your child's environment. Pay particular attention to defuzzing your child's sleeping environment (see page 126). Milk is a subtle and often overlooked allergen that may cause fluid to accumulate in the ear and breathing passages.

Treat colds early. If your child's usual pattern of cold symptoms starts with a runny nose in a happy child, progresses to a snotty nose in a cranky child, and then to a full-blown ear infection, it would be wise to consult your doctor early, before the ear infection is allowed to develop. Eustachian tube exercises (page 83) can help to pop open the ears and allow accumulated fluid to drain.

Change the situations that expose the child to colds. If your child is in day care or other situations that expose him to many other children with colds, try to make some changes. If day care is necessary, try to place your child in a less crowded environment, as much as your lifestyle and financial situation permit. A home day care set-up in which the day care provider has strict policies about sick children staying home can lessen the number of colds your child catches.

Daily medication. The use of a low-dosage, mild antibiotic daily for one to six months is a recent breakthrough in the prevention of recurrent ear infections. The antibiotic keeps the fluid that accumulates in the middle ear from becoming infected. Parents may be uneasy about using antibiotics for such a long period of time, but the daily small dose of a mild antibiotic is easier on a child's system than periodic strong antibiotics. The antibiotic that is usually used *(Gantrisin)* is the same antibiotic that some children take daily for 20 years for prevention of rheumatic fever, with no detrimental effects.

How long the child takes the antibiotic depends on the duration, frequency, and severity of the ear infections. The child's ears are examined at least once a month. In addition to looking at the child's eardrum, it is important to do a tympanogram. This test uses sound waves to detect whether or not the eardrum is moving properly. Sometimes a doctor cannot see the small amount of fluid that a tympanogram is able to detect.

We like to keep children on the prevention regimen until they have been free of ear infections and have had normal tympanograms for at least three months. Sometimes decongestants are added to the prevention regimen. In my experience decongestants do help children whose primary cause of fluid accumulation in the middle ear is allergies. In the majority of the children with recurrent ear infections decongestants do not seem to help.

This prevention regimen has many benefits. It decreases the use of stronger antibiotics to which the child may build up resistance. The Eustachian tubes may begin to function better if they are given a chance to develop unhindered by infection. Parents often notice a surge in speech development after the child has been on this regimen for a month or so, and the child's chronic irritability disappears. Finally, the regimen may prevent the need for surgery.

Surgical treatment of ear infections. Occasionally a
child will not respond to this treatment regimen for the
prevention of frequent ear infections. Fluid persists in the
middle ear and becomes thick and glue-like. It can only
be removed by opening up the eardrum (myringotomy)
and draining out the fluid. Tiny plastic tubes, about the
size of the tip of a ball-point pen, are inserted through
the eardrums to allow the accumulated fluid to drain out,
thus lessening the frequency of middle-ear infections and
producing an immediate improvement in the child's hearing. This procedure is done in the hospital or surgical center on an outpatient basis, under anesthesia. It takes about
20 minutes, and the child is usually able to go home within
an hour or two. It is important to continue the child's medical treatment and to have careful medical follow-up for
a few weeks to months afterwards, or the whole problem of ear infections may again recur. The tubes usually
stay in place for six months to a year, until they fall out
by themselves. The tiny hole left in the eardrum seals over
by itself.

Both surgical treatment and the low-dose antibiotic
regimen are ways of playing for time until your child's
immunity to germs increases and the Eustachian tubes
mature. Most children will outgrow the tendency to recurrent ear infections by age three, although ear infections
persist in some children throughout childhood.

After your child has had a few ear infections, a well-
meaning friend or relative may suggest that you take the
child to an ear specialist. The specialist is a surgeon,
trained primarily in the surgical management of ear problems. He or she does not have the advantage of seeing
your child over a period of months or years. It is better
to stick with your child's primary physician who treats
ear infections primarily with medication and is less likely
to recommend a more radical remedy like surgery. If your
doctor thinks surgery would be beneficial, he or she will
refer you to a specialist, and both doctors will decide together if surgery is necessary. Your child will be better
off for the extra care and communication.

Swimmer's Ear

The lining of the ear canal, outside of the eardrum, can also become infected. This is called **otitis externa**. The lining of the ear canal contains glands which normally secrete a protective waxy coating. This lining is water repellant and contains secretions too acidic for the survival of invading germs. An external ear infection occurs when this protective lining is broken down. Prolonged contact with water, as with swimming, may wash away the protective coating of the ear canal and provide a warm moist environment for the invasion of germs. Irritation of the ear canal may also occur from over-zealous wax removal with objects such as cotton swabs and bobbypins. My grandfather used to tell us, "Never put anything smaller than your elbow in your ear." That was wise advice.

How to recognize an outer ear infection.   Outer ear infections usually occur during the swimming season; middle ear infections tend to occur during the winter, when colds are more common. Here's what to look for in an outer ear infection:

Your child's ear canal itches and rapidly becomes painful.

Pulling on the earlobe or pressing upward behind it is painful.

The child doesn't want his ear touched.

Hearing is usually not affected, unless the infection also involves the eardrum or the ear canal is plugged with wax or drainage.

Treatment.   An outer ear infection is usually treated with ear drops which contain cortisone to control the itching and swelling of the ear canal, an antibiotic to treat the infection, and a topical anesthetic to ease the pain. It may be difficult for your doctor to treat this type of ear infection without seeing your child, since he or she cannot be sure of the severity or location of the infection.

Tips on applying ear drops. Instruct your child to lie on his side with the infected ear upward. Gently pull the auricle (the outer rim of the ear) up and back to straighten the ear canal and allow the drops to flow deeper into the canal. Insert the drops, then gently pump on the ear cartilage just above the earlobe to massage the drops further down into the canal. If the canal is plugged with wax or drainage, your doctor may need to clean out the debris in order for the drops to reach the infected lining of the canal. If the canals are very swollen and the drops won't stay in, your doctor may place a small, ear-drop saturated gauze wick into the canal. This allows the drops to penetrate more deeply. If the infection is also in the eardrum, your doctor may prescribe an oral antibiotic.

How to prevent external ear infections. Show your child how to tilt and shake his head to one side after swimming to encourage the water to drain out of the ear canals by gravity. Roll a small piece of tissue between your thumb and forefinger and gently insert it a short distance into the canal in order to absorb the remaining water. If your child swims frequently, squirt ear drops into your child's ears immediately after cleaning the water out. You can use either a prescription ear drop from your doctor or make your own. A mild acidic solution such as white vinegar diluted with an equal amount of water is very effective. Using ear plugs while swimming may irritate the lining of the ear canal and actually increase the risk of external ear infection. They should not be used without your doctor's advice.

Don't put any irritating objects into the ear to scratch the itch or to clean out wax. Unless the wax causes pain or interferes with your child's hearing it is wise to leave it alone. If earwax is a problem, consult your doctor for appropriate methods of removing it. Here is one method tor to soften the wax *(Cerumenex or Debrox)*. Be sure to use these drops only as directed and remove them within 30 minutes after use. After the wax has been softened, gently irrigate the ear canal using a Water Pik on a low setting. I use this method in the office quite frequently. If your child is not familiar with the Water Pik show him first how it is used on teeth. When set on low the jet of water will not cause pain, but it may initially startle your child if he is not properly prepared. Never attempt to remove wax from your child's ear if you suspect he has an underlying middle ear infection.

Sinus Infections

Sinusitis is one of the most commonly overlooked and under-treated respiratory infections in childhood. Unlike earaches or sore throats, the symptoms of sinus infections may be very subtle and easily missed.

The sinuses are small cavities in the facial bones along the side of the nose, beneath the eyes, between the eyes, and above the eyebrows. The lining of the sinuses becomes inflamed during a cold and secretes mucus similar to that found in the nose. Usually, as a cold heals, the fluid which accumulates in the sinuses drains out through openings into the nose. Occasionally the fluid stays in the sinuses, and the sinuses become filled with secretions. During a cold it is easy to remove secretions from the nose by blowing it; however, you cannot clear out the sinuses this way. Sometimes the fluid stays in the sinuses and eventually becomes infected. When a cold lingers on more than a week or two, it usually means a sinus infection is developing.

How to Recognize Sinus Infections
When should you suspect that your child is developing a sinus infection? Here are some signs to watch for:

A cold that lingers on more than a week or two

Dark circles under the eyes and puffy lower eyelids, caused by congestion in the veins along the sinuses

A pale, puffy, peaked face

A thick, yellow discharge from the nose and/or eyes

A productive cough, usually worse at night

A tickling sensation in the throat, especially at night, caused by the sinuses draining into the throat.

The child may also have a low-grade fever and very odorous breath coming from the infected mucus in the back of the throat. He may complain of headaches just above and between the eyes. Sometimes it hurts to press on the sinuses above and below the eyes and alongside the nose.

It is important to remember that the child may not act or appear very sick with a sinus infection. The younger the child, the more subtle the symptoms. Sinuses begin to be large enough to be easily infected around the age of two or three years. Parents should watch for sinus infections in the child who has experienced frequent colds and ear infections during the first year or two, who seems to outgrow the ear infections around the third year, but who has colds that linger on for a long time. Parents often tell me that these children are tired a lot, look peaked, are even willing to take afternoon naps. Chronic fatigue during and following a cold is one of the most common symptoms of sinus infections in adolescents. Allergic children are particularly prone to sinus infections. Any child whose cold lingers on longer than ten days, is peaked, tired, coughing, and just doesn't seem well should be examined by your doctor for a possible sinus infection.

Treating Sinus Infections
The things you do to clear a sinus infection are basically the same things you do to treat colds and ear infections, but it takes more intense and more persistent treatment.

Humidity.   As with the treatment of nose and chest congestion, your goal is to keep the secretions thin and moving. A warm shower three or four times a day and a vaporizer at night can help to loosen sinus congestion. Sinus infections are particularly common during allergy season and during the winter months of dry central heating.

Good nasal hygiene.   Children tend to be sniffers, not blowers. Encourage your child to blow his nose gently and not sniff the secretions back up into the sinuses. Noseblowing is particularly effective during warm showers.

Decongestants and nose drops may be effective if allergies are the cause of fluid accumulation in the sinuses. Decongestants may thicken the secretions and slow down their draining into the nose, but if there is profuse nasal congestion accompanying the sinus inflammation, nose drops may be effective in opening the passages from the sinuses into the nose. Avoid respiratory irritants such as cigarette smoke and dust. Antihistamines may be used during allergy season.

Antibiotics.   Infections that are enclosed within bones are more difficult to treat with antibiotics. This is true of sinus infections. It is not unusual for a child to need four to six weeks of antibiotics to completely clear up a sinus infection. After seven to ten days of antibiotic treatment the child may seem better, but may not be completely well.

Sinus irrigation.   In sinus infections that are particularly resistant to treatment, your doctor may need to wash out the sinuses. He does this by placing a small tube into the passage between the nose and the sinuses and flushing them out. This is very effective in the older child and adolescent, although it is somewhat uncomfortable. Younger children usually will not tolerate this procedure.

Sore Throats

The medical term for a sore throat is **pharyngitis**, inflammation of the pharynx or throat. There are two types of sore throats, viral and bacterial. When your doctor examines your child, he or she tries to determine if the sore throat is caused by a virus or by bacteria.

Throats infected by viruses may hurt a lot, but look normal when the doctor examines them. Some virus infections of the throat are accompanied by tiny painful ulcers on the roof of the mouth and on the inside of the cheeks. This is called **herpangina**. This type of infection is similar, but not identical to the virus that causes cold sores on the lips. In viral throat infections the glands beneath the jaw are usually not as swollen as they are with bacterial infections. Headaches and muscle aches often accompany viral sore throats. There may be a fever, but it tends to be minimal or, if very high, tends to go up and down with the use of fever-lowering medication. Sometimes your doctor may need to take a throat culture to determine whether your child's throat infection is caused by a virus or bacteria. Viral sore throats subside without antibiotics; bacterial sore throats need antibiotic treatment.

Treating Sore Throats

Older children can gargle with salt water to relieve some of the discomfort of a sore throat. Analgesic sprays or throat lozenges may also be soothing. Since it may hurt to swallow, clear fluids and soft foods may be the only things that your child can eat. In certain types of viral sore throats (for example, herpangina), acidic fluids such as orange juice may be irritating; this characteristic can help to identify a viral infection.

Viral sore throats, like the common cold, are most contagious on the day before and during the first few days of the illness. They are only minimally contagious toward the end of the time the child has symptoms.

Bacterial sore throats.   The usual culprit in a bacterial sore throat is the bacteria streptococcus. With a bacterial sore throat a child appears and acts much sicker than with a viral sore throat. Although the fever may not be very high (usually around 102 °F), it does not come down easily with fever-lowering medication. The child with a strep throat appears generally ill and may have other symptoms as well: vomiting, abdominal pain, joint aches, rapid heartbeat, and lethargy. He may want to do nothing but rest. When your doctor examines the child the throat may look normal and a throat culture may be necessary to make the diagnosis. Usually, however, the throat has a characteristic beefy red appearance, the tonsils are swollen and are covered with a white, odorous secretion, and the glands in back of the jaw are very swollen and tender. Strep throat is unusual in the child under two, but it does occur. It is more common in the school-age child and adolescent. Usually, the child with strep throat becomes progressively more sick if left untreated.

Sometimes a rash may appear with strep throat; this is called **scarlet fever**. Scarlet fever is nothing more than strep throat with a rash and is no more serious. The rash is the result of a toxin released into the blood stream by the streptococcus bacteria. It looks very much like a sunburn over the cheeks and trunk, but it is not present around the mouth—the child may look as if he has a white mustache.

Treating bacterial sore throats.   Antibiotics are necessary to treat bacterial sore throats. If the diagnosis is streptococcus, penicillin is given for ten days. Because strep throat is very contagious, it may be wise to treat all the children in the family, as well as other close contacts, to prevent them from spreading the disease at school or among their friends. They should be put on half the treatment dose of penicillin for five days. The incubation period for strep throat is four to seven days. After 24 hours of antibiotic treatment, your child is no longer contagious.

Why it is important to treat strep throat. Doctors'
offices now have throat culture kits which give results
within five minutes. Undiagnosed or untreated strep
throat may lead to rheumatic fever and consequent damage to the heart or kidneys. Fortunately, with improved
awareness, better diagnostic techniques, and easier access
to medical care, rheumatic fever is no longer a common
disease.

Croup

Croup is a cough that sounds like a "seal bark." It is caused
by inflammation and swelling of the vocal cords and adjacent windpipe or trachea. Because the swelling of the
vocal cords may obstruct the passage of air, croup is potentially a very serious respiratory infection. Croup is usually
caused by viruses similar to those that cause the common
cold, but it may occasionally be caused by a bacterial infection. It is contracted in the same way as the common
cold, from airborne droplets from the cough or sneezing
of another child. Croup is most common in the winter.
    Croup may begin suddenly at night with the child sit-
ting up in bed barking like a seal, or it may begin gradually with cold symptoms which turn into a croupy cough
over two or three nights. The main goal in taking care of
the child with croup is to recognize when it is serious and
when it is not.

Signs of Non-Serious Croup
If your child's cough sounds croupy, but he is smiling,
happy, and playful and is not having trouble breathing,
he probably has nothing more than a noisy cold. In fact,
generally speaking, the noisier the child, the less serious
the respiratory infection. It takes a lot of air to produce
all that sound, and if your child is moving a lot of air in
and out, the obstruction is not serious. Also, if your child
is able to sleep without too much disruption, it is unlikely
that the croup is serious.

Watching your child in action may give you a clue as to the seriousness of the breathing obstruction. If the child is sitting up in bed or on the floor, is interested in the persons and things in his environment, and does not seem to be as bothered about the whole affair as you are, then you do not have to worry. Children who are developing a serious respiratory problem seem to tune out their environment and tune in to themselves, as if they need to concentrate all their attention and energy on getting enough air. Children don't panic, they just become quiet. And they are right. Croup should be treated with concern but not panic.

Signs of Serious Croup
More serious croup infections can keep your child from being able to get enough air. These are the signs of serious croup:

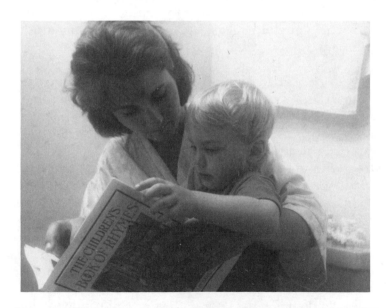

A calming story and a steamy bathroom
relieve symptoms of croup.

The throat caves in at the front of the neck just above the breast bone when the child takes a breath. This is called **indrawing**.

There is increasingly labored, noisy breathing (called **stridor**), mainly during inhalation.

The child seems anxious, restless, or even panicky.

If your child is showing signs of serious croup, try the following measures. If there is no improvement, seek medical attention immediately.

Treating Your Child's Croup
Anxiety aggravates breathing difficulties. You may have to use all your parental ingenuity to calm your child. Settle him in bed or on your lap. Place him upright, at about a 45-degree angle, using pillows. Read him a story, play soft music, or let him watch a soothing program on television. Sleep is one of the best therapies for croup. If you can help your child fall asleep, the indrawing and stridor will usually decrease.

Humidity. High humidity helps to relieve croup symptoms. Use a cool mist vaporizer in the bedroom with the doors closed. You can make a homemade croup tent by covering your child's crib with a sheet and placing the vaporizer near an opening in the sheet. Sometimes children with croup do not want to be left alone in bed. If this is the case sit your child on your lap with his head against your shoulder while the steam from the vaporizer rises toward his nose and mouth. Sing to him, trying to get him off to sleep.

Another way to create a humid environment is to take your child into the bathroom, turn on the hot water in the shower, sink, and tub, and close the doors and windows. Sit down on the floor with your child and read him a story. Or put a pillow against the wall to help him sit upright while leaning his head against you. Allow him to breathe the heavy steam for at least 20 minutes. This will often help a croupy child settle down and fall asleep.

Other suggestions. Do not give your croupy child over-the-counter medicines without your doctor's advice, especially decongestants. These may dry out the breathing passages and aggravate the croup. Because croup is usually caused by a virus, antibiotics are not usually necessary. A low-grade fever (100° to 101 °F) may be present, and your child may benefit from fever-lowering medications.

Give your child plenty of fluids. Children with breathing difficulties seldom eat much, but they should drink frequently and slowly; small sips through a straw work well. Large, sudden gulps may cause vomiting.

If your child is breastfeeding, encourage him to nurse during an attack of croup. Breastfeeding will provide him with nutritious fluids and will help him relax. I recently had to hospitalize an 18-month-old boy for treatment of severe croup. The mother periodically leaned over the crib rail and lifted up the side of the croup tent to breastfeed. After a minute or two of nursing, he would settle down, and the stridor almost ceased.

Croup is usually worse at night. If you can parent your child through the nighttime breathing difficulty, daytime often brings relief. If you are uncertain about the severity of your child's croup or are not sure that your home treatment is working, call your doctor or take your child to the hospital. It is all right to take your child outdoors. Many children actually improve on their way to the hospital or doctor's office because of the higher humidity outside.

Epiglottitis

Epiglottitis is a rapidly progressing, life-threatening, croup-like illness caused by inflammation of the epiglottis, the tissue about the size of a thumbnail just above the entrance to the windpipe. Epiglottitis can completely obstruct the airway; it is a serious medical emergency needing immediate treatment.

Unlike croup, which is caused by a virus, epiglottitis is caused by bacteria. Epiglottitis usually occurs in a child over three years of age. The temperature is high (103°F or above), and the child looks and acts very sick. The child with epiglottitis will sit up in bed with his mouth wide open and behave as if he is choking. He is often unable to swallow his saliva and will drool. He produces a prolonged hoarse, droning-type of sound as he inhales each breath. He may not have any difficulty exhaling. It may seem as if something is caught on the back of his tongue, and the child's tongue often protrudes forward with each breath, as if he is trying to further open the passage. The child with epiglottitis does not respond to the treatment outlined for croup.

If you suspect epiglottitis, call your doctor immediately or take your child immediately to the nearest hospital. The treatment at the hospital will consist mainly of antibiotics and high humidity. Most likely, a tube will need to be inserted through the child's nose or mouth into his throat to allow air to pass the obstruction.

Bronchitis

Bronchitis is an inflammation of the bronchi, the lower airways which branch out from the end of the windpipe into the lungs. Infection or allergy may inflame the lining of the bronchi, causing mucus to be secreted into the breathing passages and the muscles in the walls of the bronchi to go into spasms. This narrows the bronchial passages, causing wheezing and indrawing (caving-in of the chest wall between the ribs during inhalation). Breathing is usually labored during bronchitis since it takes more effort to move air through these narrowed passages.

How to Recognize Bronchitis

A productive, somewhat musical cough accompanies bronchitis. The child wheezes when exhaling, and there is indrawing when he inhales. His temperature may be normal, or he may have a low-grade fever if the infection is caused by a virus. If it is a bacterial infection, the fever will be higher (102° or 103 °F). As with croup, the severity of bronchitis depends on how much your child is bothered by it.

If your child wheezes only during exhalation, when the airways are narrowest, but has no trouble during inhalation (no indrawing), it is much less serious than if he experiences breathing difficulty with both. If your child looks like a "happy wheezer"—he is generally happy, but breathing very noisily—there is less reason to be concerned about the bronchitis. Beware of the happy wheezer who becomes progressively more tired. Some children can wheeze for a couple of days without apparent difficulty, but gradually they become tired and exhausted. At that point, breathing difficulties can rapidly become more serious.

At-Home Help for Bronchitis
Calming and comforting the child and placing him in a humid environment will help to relieve bronchitis sym-

---

Danger Signs in a Child with Breathing Difficulties

Seek immediate medical attention when any of these symptoms appear in a child who is having difficulty breathing:

The child has a persistent fever of 103°F or more.

The child persistently leans forward to breathe and drools because he cannot swallow his saliva.

The child appears to be very sick in addition to having difficulty breathing.

The indrawing and stridor are becoming worse.

The child's breathing rate is more than sixty breaths per minute.

The lips and fingernails are becoming blue or dusky.

The child is not responding to humidity and attempts to calm him.

ptoms. Use a vaporizer or turn on the shower in the bathroom and sit with your child in the steam. To help your child cough up the mucus, use the chest physiotherapy technique described on pages 101-102.

Unless advised by your doctor, do not give your child antihistamines or decongestants as these thicken the secretions and make them more difficult to cough up. Expectorant-type cough medicines may be used, since these thin the secretions and make them easier to clear from the airways.

Seek medical attention for a child with bronchitis when the following signs occur:

The child has a fever of 102°F or higher.

The child's breathing becomes progressively more difficult.

There are signs of bacterial infections: high fever, snotty nose and draining eyes, thick yellow sputum being coughed up from the lungs, rapid heart rate.

The cough is bothering the child, particularly at night.

The child is becoming progressively more tired and exhausted from coughing and wheezing.

Pneumonia

Pneumonia sounds very serious; the term had dreadful implications in grandmother's day. I usually use the term lung infection when explaining this illness to parents. Pneumonia is an infection of the tissue in the lowest parts of the airways, at the very end of the bronchi. Sometimes the bronchi are also infected; this is called bronchiopneumonia. Modern antibiotics have taken much of the fear out of having pneumonia. It is not at all the serious lung condition it used to be.

A few days of cold symptoms precede the onset of pneumonia. Other symptoms are a high fever (103°F or above), a severe cough that produces thick yellow mucus (children often swallow the mucus as soon as they cough it up, so you may not see it), and a rapid heart beat. The child seems listless and just wants to lie in bed. The fever associated with untreated bacterial pneumonia is difficult to bring down with fever-lowering medication. The fever of a cold or viral chest infection goes down rapidly when it is treated.

Treating Pneumonia

Your doctor must decide whether the pneumonia is caused by bacteria or a virus. With viral pneumonia, a child coughs profusely, and the cough lingers on a while. The fever may be low or high, but it is easy to control. The child does not seem to be particularly sick and is not getting worse. With bacterial pneumonia the fever stays high, the child appears to be very ill, the heartbeat is rapid, and the general condition of the child worsens each day. When examining your child's chest, the doctor listens for sounds characteristic of certain types of pneumonia and also tries to pinpoint the location of the infection. Your doctor may order a chest x-ray to clarify the diagnosis at the time of the first office visit and again at the end of the illness to be sure that the chest is completely clear. Sometimes the diagnosis is obvious, and a chest x-ray may not be necessary.

Bacterial pneumonia is treated with antibiotics. If a child is very sick the doctor may choose to hospitalize him in order to give him intravenous antibiotics. If your child is vomiting and cannot keep down oral antibiotics, your doctor may choose to give him one or two initial doses by injection; he can take oral antibiotics when the vomiting subsides.

At-home treatment for pneumonia. Your doctor can mark the location of the pneumonia on your child's chest and show you how to clap on his back and chest to help loosen secretions in the lungs. To do this **chest physiotherapy** place your child on your lap or on a bed, with a heavy shirt or towel over the affected area. With your hand cupped, vigorously clap over the area with pneumonia for at least a minute or two, four or more times a day. Clap hard enough to encourage your child to cough but not hard enough to cause pain. Children are seldom bothered by this chest physiotherapy.

Give your child plenty of fluids to help loosen the secretions. Children often do not want to eat when they have pneumonia (it may trigger vomiting), but they need fluids. Small sips very frequently are the best way to get the fluids into the child without causing vomiting.

Use the fever-lowering measures outlined in Chapter Four. Use cough medicines wisely and only as directed by your doctor. With pneumonia it is wise to limit the use of cough syrup since you want your child to cough up the infected mucus. Cough looseners (expectorants) can be used during the day, with a cough suppressant added at night.

CHAPTER 6

Common Intestinal Problems

All children have occasional bouts with diarrhea, constipation, spitting-up, and tummy aches while they're growing up. Most are mild and pass quickly. If you know what
to watch for and how to help when your child is having
problems in her digestive system, you can help her feel
better and prevent things from getting worse.

Normal Variations in Bowel Habits

It stands to reason that a child's stool may be as variable
as her diet, since bowel movements are made up in large
part of the residue of undigested food. If you change what
goes into the mouth, what comes out the other end will
also change. There are plenty of common, normal varia-
tions in the stools and bowel habits of infants and children. Stools of breastfed babies tend to be more frequent,
looser, and mustard yellow in color. Formula-fed infants

have stools which are firmer, greenish-brown, less frequent, and smellier. Iron-containing foods or formulas normally produce a darker, greenish stool. An occasional green stool in a healthy infant is of no consequence. Mucus swallowed during teething will often produce a loose, mucousy stool. Frequency of bowel movements varies considerably in children and infants, from one or two a day (more in newborns) to one every three or four days.

Expect diarrhea during and following antibiotic therapy. Anything which produces acidic stools (antibiotics, allergies, diets with lots of acid) may also bring a red bottom, since the acid irritates the skin. Bowel changes that signal serious intestinal problems are usually accompanied by other obvious signs such as weight loss, abdominal pain, fever, or anemia. Most bowel changes in children are well within the realm of normal.

Constipation

Constipation refers to the consistency of stools and the difficulty in passing them, not to the frequency of bowel movements. Some infants and small children normally have bowel movements only once every three to five days. If your child does not appear uncomfortable, she is not constipated. If your infant's bowel movements are three to four days apart (or longer), but are reasonably soft and are passed without difficulty, she is not constipated. A constipated infant draws her legs up onto her abdomen and becomes red in the face as she strains to pass hard pellet-like stools. Since the infant's rectum is often small, the passage of a hard stool may cause a small tear in the wall of the rectum. This is called a **rectal fissure.** It may produce a few streaks of fresh blood in the stool or a few drops of blood on the diaper. Rectal fissures can start a vicious cycle of constipation in an infant. Because it hurts to pass a hard stool past this tear, the baby may voluntarily hold onto the stool, creating more constipation. If your infant or child has a rectal fissure, apply a small amount of glycerine over the area to soothe it and ease the passage of the stool. Persistently black, tarry, or bloody stools indicate bleeding in the intestines. Notify your doctor if this occurs.

Treating Constipation

Long-term constipation takes at least four to six weeks to treat. Constipation stretches your child's intestines, and it may take four to six weeks of diet changes to treat the problem.

Constipation in infants. Totally breastfed babies are rarely constipated, although after the newborn stage they may go several days or a week between stools. Constipation can be a problem in babies who have started solids and in formula-fed infants.

Rice cereal, bananas, apples, and carrots are all constipating foods. Stay away from these if constipation is a problem for your baby. Instead, encourage her to eat foods that have a laxative effect: prunes, pears, apricots, peaches.

Babies usually accept diluted prune juice; start with one tablespoon a day and work up to eight ounces. Your baby might like prune puree, or you may have to disguise it by mixing the strained prunes with another favorite food. Try to give your constipated infant two to three tablespoons of strained prunes daily.

Offer your child water frequently between meals, or if exclusively formula-fed, between feedings. Smaller, more frequent feedings may also help to lessen constipation in a formula-fed infant. You may want to experiment with different kinds of formula to see if another type makes bowel movements easier. Too much cow's milk may also produce constipation (or diarrhea).

Adding fiber to your infant's diet will help with constipation. Fiber softens the stools by drawing water into them. It also adds bulk to the stools, which makes them pass more quickly through your child's intestines. Bran cereals, graham crackers, and other whole-grain breads and crackers are good sources of fiber for babies.

When your infant is having difficulty passing a stool, insert a glycerine suppository or liquid glycerine in a dropper high into her rectum. (These are available at drug stores without a prescription.) This is especially helpful if she has a rectal fissure. Glycerine suppositories look like little rocket ships. For the tiny baby you may have to cut the suppository in half and insert only the pointed top end. Hold the baby's buttocks together for a few minutes so that the glycerine will dissolve.

If diet changes are not effective in resolving your baby's constipation, your doctor may recommend a stool softener such as *Colase, Maltsupex,* or *Metamucil.* Mineral oil, one tablespoon a day until the stools soften, may also be helpful.

Constipation in the older child.   In addition to the kinds of diet changes suggested above for infants, the older child needs some other measures to resolve constipation since she can now choose whether or not to respond to the urge to defecate. Sometimes older children who are chronically constipated will soil their pants. This is not diarrhea; the child is still constipated. The soiling is due to the leaking of stools from the lower intestinal muscles which have been weakened by chronic constipation. This child requires intensive and long-term treatment of her constipation.

Introduce your young child to the toilet gradually, without pressure, so that she does not fear having a bowel movement and decide to hold on to her productions. Children are ready for toilet-training at different ages, so respect your child's cues. Teach your child to respond immediately to the urge-to-go signal and not to hold on to her stools. Explain that not paying attention to the signal weakens the "doughnut muscles" around the rectum and that this will eventually cause her to have pain when she has a bowel movement. Tell her to "go when you have to go."

In addition to the high-fiber foods mentioned above for infants, your older child's diet should include fiber in the form of green leafy vegetables and raw fruits. Potentially constipating foods in the older child include rice, cheese, bananas, and chocolate. Encourage the older child to drink lots of liquids, at least four eight-ounce glasses of water daily.

In addition to the stool-softeners mentioned above, laxatives may be used for the older child. Sometimes prescription laxatives may also be necessary. If the above measures fail to produce normal stooling habits, you may need to start your child's treatment regimen with a clean slate by giving her an enema.

How to give an enema.　In babies, use a Fleet enema specially formulated for infants. Apply petroleum jelly to the tip of the syringe. Gently insert the tip into the baby's rectum (as you do with a thermometer), allowing it to seek its own path. Then squeeze gently. Remove the syringe and hold the baby's buttocks together. Give the enema three to five minutes to work before you let go.

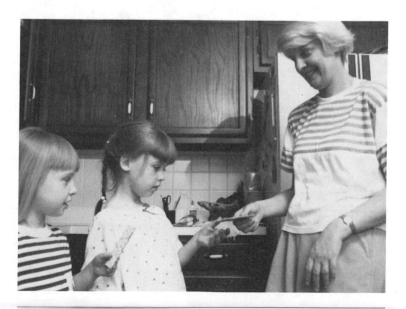

Whole-grain crackers provide fiber, which prevents constipation.

In the child over three, you can use an adult-type Fleet enema. For a thirty-to-sixty-pound child use half a dose; over sixty-pounds, use a full dose. Place your child on her side and flex her upper leg toward her abdomen. After you have inserted the enema hold the buttocks together for ten minutes, if possible, and then place your child on the toilet. An enema can be repeated after an hour if necessary.

Diarrhea

Diarrhea means "liquid stools" and refers more to the consistency of the stools than to the frequency. The most common causes of diarrhea in infancy and childhood are colds, antibiotic therapy, food intolerance, and gastrointestinal infections.

The most frequent cause of problem diarrhea in infants and children is an intestinal infection called **gastroenteritis.** This is usually caused by a virus. When the intestinal lining becomes infected it heals very slowly. During the healing process the enzymes in the intestinal lining that help digest and absorb food do not function properly. The result is stools that are very frequent, watery, explosive, green, mucousy, and foul-smelling. This kind of diarrhea is usually accompanied by cold symptoms. The child seems generally sick.

Diarrhea becomes a worrisome problem when it leads to dehydration, the result of your child losing more water and body salts through her stools than she is taking in. Your child's body contains a balance of water and salts (called electrolytes). A proper balance is necessary for organs to functions. Diarrhea stools cause the body to lose water and electrolytes. Vomiting in addition to having diarrhea increases the likelihood of dehydration. Signs of dehydration are:

Obvious weight loss

Dry eyes, dry skin, and dry mouth

Diminishing urine output

An increasingly quiet, lethargic child

Loose, wrinkled skin

Fever

If there is no weight loss with childhood diarrhea, then there is no problem. No matter how frequent and loose your child's stools seem to be, if she is happy, bright-eyed, and not showing signs of dehydration, you do not have to worry.

Management and Treatment of Diarrhea

Your main goal in treating your child's diarrhea is to avoid dehydration. Try to determine whether the diarrhea is just a nuisance or whether it is severe enough to cause dehydration. Use the signs listed above to recognize dehydration. You will need to cut back on those foods in your child's diet that cannot be absorbed by infected intestines and give her more of those things which contain the extra water and minerals which she has lost. The following is a step-by-step approach.

Weigh your baby or child. Using the most accurate scale you can obtain, weigh your baby or child, naked, as soon as she starts vomiting or having diarrhea. This is her baseline weight. Weigh her daily, preferably each morning before you feed her, and record the weight. If your child has no significant weight loss, she is not becoming dehydrated. If your child loses five percent of her baseline body weight (for example, a weight loss of one pound in a twenty-pound child) she has experienced a significant amount of dehydration, and you should call your doctor immediately. Rapid weight loss is of more concern than a gradual weight loss. A twenty-pound infant who loses a pound of body weight over a period of two days is of much greater concern than one who loses the same amount of weight over a period of two weeks. Infants usually appear very sick if they are losing weight rapidly; they do not act as sick if the weight loss has been gradual.

Stop all solid foods, dairy products, and formulas made with cow's milk. If you are breastfeeding, it is rarely necessary to stop even temporarily, since human milk is not as irritating to infected intestines as cow's milk products and may even be therapeutic. Oftentimes a breastfeeding infant will only take breast milk during a bout of vomiting or diarrhea and will wisely refuse any other foods or liquids. During a recent flu epidemic I noticed that the breastfed infants seemed to recover faster and to experience less dehydration and hospitalization than did formula-fed infants.

Give your child a clear fluid diet. Your basic goal is to replace at one end the fluid that your child is losing at the other. The fluids listed below are easy to digest and provide the calories and salts which your child needs to replace those lost with diarrhea:

Oral electrolyte solutions *(Pedialyte, Lytren)*. These are available at your pharmacy or grocery store without prescription. Do not use these electrolyte solutions for more than 24 hours without checking with your physician.

Flat ginger ale and colas. Place these solutions in a flat wide pan to allow the bubbles to evaporate.

A sugar solution prepared by adding one tablespoon of ordinary table sugar to eight ounces of boiled water. (Do not boil the sugar solution because boiling may cause the water to evaporate and make the solution too strong.) This solution may be used at night when the other solutions are not easily available. However, sugar solutions do not contain the electrolytes which your child needs.

Small, frequent feedings (two ounces at a time for infants) are best. A good rule of thumb is to give half as much twice as often. Use the "sips and chips" method to provide fluids to the older child. Make your own ginger-ale, cola, or oral-electrolyte-solution popsicles and let your child suck on these and ice chips all day long. Popsicles provide a steady flow of fluid that resembles the steady drip of intravenous treatment. This clear fluid diet should not be continued more than forty-eight hours without checking with your doctor, since clear fluids alone continued for too long may themselves produce a kind of diarrhea called "starvation stools."

After twenty-four to forty-eight hours, add semisolid food. As your child's stools become more solid, so can the diet. If your child is not losing weight and the diarrhea has lessened somewhat, you can add foods such as rice cereal without milk or mashed bananas to her diet. Also continue the regimen of small, frequent fluid feedings. As the stools continue to improve gradually add applesauce, saltine crackers, toast, gelatin, mashed potatoes, and plain yogurt. The BRAT diet (bananas, rice, applesauce, and unbuttered toast) is a time-tested favorite.

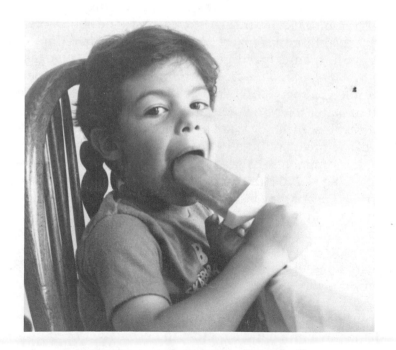

Popsicles replace fluids lost with diarrhea.

Resume milk or formula feedings very gradually. Formula or cow's milk should not return to your child's diet until you have seen much improvement in the diarrhea, usually around day three. On the first day of giving formula, dilute the already mixed formula with an equal part of boiled water (half-strength formula). The next day use three-quarter strength (three parts prepared formula to one part boiled water), and the next day resume giving full-strength milk or formula. Do not boil milk or give undiluted skim milk to a child who has diarrhea since these solutions are too concentrated and may worsen the dehydration.

If the diarrhea worsens after resuming dairy products, go back a few steps in the regimen and begin again. If your child's intestinal infection has been severe enough, there may be temporary damage to the lining of the intestines, and there may be insufficient amounts of the enzyme lactase, which is necessary for digesting milk. For this reason a lactose-free soy formula may be better tolerated than formulas made with cow's milk. Sometimes a hypoallergenic predigested formula *(Nutramigen, Pregestamil, Carnation Good Start, Alimentum)* may be better tolerated by your child's healing intestines. Yogurt is often better tolerated than milk or milk-based formulas. Lactase insufficiency is not a problem in breastfed infants because breast milk is better tolerated than formula.

It is common to have a prolonged period of loose stools following an intestinal infection. I call this "nuisance diarrhea," and it may last for several weeks or months. The intestinal lining is very slow to heal in most children. If your child has persistent diarrhea, it is more important to focus on the total child than on her bottom. If she appears generally well and is not continuing to lose weight, you do not need to worry, even if her stools remain loose.

Treating the sore bottom. It is common for an infant's diaper area or a child's bottom to become very red during a diarrhea episode. This is because infected stools are often very acidic and irritate the skin. This acid "burn" may be prevented by using a zinc-oxide barrier cream wit each diaper change and changing the child's diapers a promptly as possible. Soaking in a baking soda bath (cne tablespoon of baking soda to a couple inches of water) is also soothing. Diarrhea is often spread by contact. It is very important to wash your hands thoroughly following diaper changes.

Medications for diarrhea. In general, diarrhea is best treated with diet restrictions and fluid replacement rather than with drugs. However, some over-the-counter medications are safe and sometimes effective in children. Acidophilus capsules may help restore the normal bacteria in the gut (the good bacteria that keep the harmful bacteria under control) and lessen the diarrhea. These capsules are available in health food stores. Children one to three years of age should take one to three capsules a day.

Imodium is a safe and effective over-the-counter antidiarrheal medication. The dosage is listed on the package.

Narcotic medications, which are often used to control diarrhea in adults, are generally not safe for children. These medications stop the diarrhea by slowing down the action of the intestines. This allows the germs and infected fluid to stagnate in the gut and increases the chance of these germs entering the child's bloodstream where they can cause serious illness.

When to Call Your Doctor about Diarrhea

If you have tried the measures listed above but your child continues to lose weight, shows signs of dehydration, has increasing abdominal pain, or looks increasingly ill, call your doctor for more advice. Before making your call have the following information available:

The frequency of stools and what they look like

How much weight loss in how much time

Any associated symptoms such as fever, a cold, indi-
cations of dehydration

Presence and frequency of vomiting

What kind of treatment you have been giving.

Vomiting

Spitting-Up in Young Infants

Most vomiting in the first three months is simply
regurgitation—spitting up resulting from a temporary feeding problem, such as swallowing air or eating too much.
It is normal for infants to spit up once or twice a day. Some
healthy babies gain weight normally even though they spit
up six to ten times a day. You can often spot the parents
of a "spitter" by the dried milk on the shoulders of their
clothing. (If your baby spits up a lot, wear prints and stay
away from dark colors. And keep a cloth diaper handy
wherever you go.) This type of vomiting is more of a laundry problem than a medical problem and usually subsides
without treatment over the next few months. If your baby
is gaining weight well and experiencing no abdominal discomfort during the spitting-up then you do not need to
worry.

Causes of spitting-up

Some babies, formula- and breastfed, gulp down their milk
like little barracudas and don't know when to stop. Tiny
babies have tiny tummies which if over-filled will rebel.
Vomiting or explosive diarrhea immediately after the feeding are signs of over-feeding. If you are formula-feeding,
give your child smaller more frequent feedings. If breastfeeding, stop and burp your baby and settle her down for
a few minutes as you switch sides.

Overeager eaters tend to swallow a lot of air along with
their milk. The air settles beneath the food in the stomach. When the stomach contracts, the air acts as a pneu-
matic pump and pushes some of the milk back up the
esophagus and all over the parent. Burping can help to

prevent this. Formula-fed babies who tend to spit up should be burped after every three ounces of milk. Breastfed babies who tend to spit up should be burped when switching sides. If your breastfed baby nurses longer than ten minutes on a side, take advantage of a pause in her sucking rhythm to take her off the breast and burp her after about ten minutes. You can then return her to the first breast, or switch sides.

How to burp your baby. Sit your baby on your lap. Lean her weight against the heel of your hand, placed just above her navel. This applies gentle pressure to the abdomen. Firmly pat or rub the baby's back.

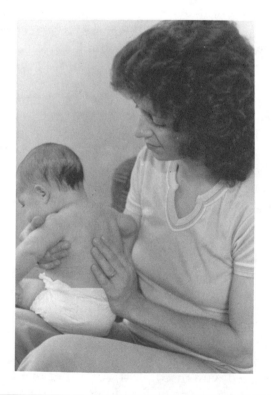

Frequent burping prevents spitting-up. Burp your baby on your lap with your hand against his abdomen.

Keep your baby in an upright position for as long as you can after each feeding. Gravity will help to hold the milk down. If you can't hold your baby after a feeding, place her in an infant seat, tipped upward at a forty-five-degree angle or more. It takes approximately twenty minutes for breast milk to empty from the stomach and as long as an hour for formula. Excessive jostling of a baby after feeding may contribute to air-swallowing and spitting-up. Adults don't exercise after meals, and neither should babies.

Other causes of spitting-up. Milk allergy may be a cause of frequent regurgitation in the young infant. Usually, if milk allergy is the cause of spitting up, it is accompanied by other signs of discomfort: bloating, abdominal pain, colicky symptoms, diarrhea. If you are bottle-feeding, your doctor may suggest a change of formula. If you are breast-feeding, try eliminating milk and other dairy products from your diet for a week or more.

Gastroesophageal (G-E) reflux is becoming more widely recognized as a cause of regurgitation in the young infant. G-E reflux is due to a problem at the junction of the esophagus and stomach. (The esophagus is the passage between the throat and the stomach.) Normally food enters the stomach through the esophagus. When the stomach contracts, the food is pushed down into the intestines, and the junction of the esophagus and stomach closes to prevent the food from going back up into the esophagus. Sometimes the muscles around this junction malfunction and allow some milk to be refluxed back up into the esophagus.

G-E reflux usually subsides without medical treatment by six to eight months when the esophagus-stomach junction begins to function better. Sometimes G-E reflux is severe enough to hinder a baby's weight gain. Sometimes it is associated with discomfort, colic, and night-waking, since stomach acids as well as food are refluxed up into the esophagus where they irritate and cause pain. Adults call this heartburn. Parents of a baby with this problem often say, "It seems to hurt her when she spits up." The combination of regurgitation, poor weight gain, colicky symptoms, and frequent night-waking deserves medical attention. Prolonged excessive reflux of stomach acids may permanently injure the lining of the esophagus, and G-E reflux can result in a baby who is very uncomfortable and who doesn't gain weight.

If you suspect your baby has G-E reflux, give her small frequent feedings. Hold her upright during and after feedings, and burp her frequently. Consult your doctor about prescription medications.

Pyloric stenosis is one of the most serious causes of vomiting in the infant in the first month or two and requires immediate medical and surgical attention. This condition, occurring primarily in male infants between four and six weeks of age, is caused by an obstruction at the pyloris, the end of the stomach. The muscle surrounding the pyloris may be too thick to allow milk to pass easily. Milk builds up in the stomach, and the stomach swells. When the stomach muscles contract to try to force milk through the small opening, some will sneak through the partial obstruction and continue into the intestines, but some milk will be spit up through the mouth with great force. This is called projectile vomiting. If a baby is sitting on the parent's lap when projectile vomiting strikes, the milk may miss the lap entirely and hit the floor, or it may even splatter against the wall two feet away. Signs that your baby may have pyloric stenosis include:

Persistent projectile vomiting

Weight loss or failure to gain weight

Signs of dehydration: dry mouth, dry eyes, wrinkly skin, and diminished urine output

Stomach swells up like a big tense balloon after a feeding, deflates after vomiting.

Some normal healthy babies may experience projectile vomiting once or twice a day if overfed, under-burped, or jostled too much. Persistent projectile vomiting accompanied by weight loss and dehydration is cause for concern.

Pyloric stenosis may take longer to diagnose in a breastfed baby. Breastfed babies with pyloric stenosis may not become dehydrated as quickly, perhaps because breast milk may pass more easily through the obstruction.

Your doctor can usually diagnose pyloric stenosis by watching a feeding and looking for the ballooning of the tense stomach and feeling the pyloric muscle in spasm. If you suspect your infant may have pyloric stenosis, call your doctor. Do not feed your baby for an hour or two before your appointment. A baby with pyloric stenosis may need a day or two of rehydration with intravenous fluids in the hospital to correct whatever electrolyte imbalances may have been caused by dehydration. This is followed by a short surgical procedure (approximately twenty minutes). The surgeon makes a one-inch incision in the abdomen in order to open up the tight pyloric muscle. Improvement is immediate and recovery time short.

Vomiting in the Older Infant and Child

Vomiting in older babies and in children may be caused by an intestinal infection, such as intestinal flu, or it may be a sign of an underlying illness. Vomiting may be only the tip of the iceberg, especially if the child seems generally very sick. The most common serious illnesses associated with vomiting are bacterial sore throat, urinary tract infections, pneumonia, meningitis, encephalitis, and appendicitis. Here are a number of other possible causes of vomiting, listed in order of severity.

Infection. Vomiting due to intestinal infection is usually accompanied by cold symptoms, fever, abdominal pain, and diarrhea. Treatment is aimed at preventing dehydration by replacing the fluid your child is losing in the vomitus and loose diarrhea stools. Follow the diet restrictions and fluid replacement suggestions in the section on diarrhea (pages 107-110). Cool, non-carbonated drinks are best for a vomiting child. Cola that has gone flat has some anti-vomiting properties; ice chips and popsicles made with cola are effective. Anti-vomiting medications are availa ble by prescription should your child's vomiting persist and make her increasingly uncomfortable.

Food poisoning. Food poisoning symptoms usually begin a couple hours after the offending meal is eaten. Older children usually complain of the "sick to my stomach" feeling of nausea. Other signs include wretching or dry heaves and chills. There is usually no fever. The child feels sick all over and may experience some pain in the upper or mid-abdomen. Food poisoning symptoms usually subside within six to eight hours and are treated by withholding foods and giving your sick child sips of soothing liquids, ice chips, and popsicles. Explosive vomiting may produce vomitus that is blood-tinged because of a tear in the blood vessels in the lining of the esophagus. This usually is not serious and subsides quickly by giving your child cold liquids, especially ice chips and popsicles.

Intestinal obstruction. The most serious cause of vomiting in the infant and child is intestinal obstruction. Sometimes the bowel may be twisted, preventing the passage of food. Sudden onset of severe intestinal pain and projectile vomiting of green, bile-stained vomitus are signs of intestinal obstruction. The child often doubles up with pain, and her abdomen is tense and tender when you gently press on it. **Persistent green-stained vomitus, abdominal pain, and a generally unwell child require immediate medical attention. This is a medical emergency.**

*How to Communicate
with Your Doctor about Vomiting*
When phoning your doctor provide the following information:

How the vomiting started: suddenly or gradually

Frequency

Character of the vomitus: curdled, sour food or milk, clear or green

Signs of dehydration: weight loss, diminished urine output, dry eyes and mouth

Associated signs and symptoms: fever, diarrhea, headache, lethargy, stiff neck, sore throat (vomiting is common with bacterial throat infections)

Associated abdominal pain

Other household members with similar signs and symptoms

How sick your child seems to be

What treatment you have tried.

Stomach Aches

During middle childhood (six to ten years of age) at least ten percent of children experience vague types of abdominal pains. They have difficulty explaining these pains, parents have difficulty understanding them, and doctors find them hard to diagnose. These pains often subside with "tincture of time" without harming the child.

When evaluating children with these stomach pains, I am struck by one distinctive feature: they do not fit any known medical condition. Characteristics of these unexplained abdominal pains include:

Vagueness—the child cannot clearly describe the pain.

Difficulty pinpointing the site—the child usually encircles the navel with her whole hand, but can not point to the exact location of the pain.

The pain does not change; it does not become better or get any worse.

The pain does not awaken the child at night.

The pain often lessens during family holidays and summer vacations, when there is less stress.

The child is generally well.

Physical exams and laboratory tests are normal.

These unexplained abdominal pains may have a number of possible causes: constipation, food allergy or intolerance (especially to dairy products); tense, high-strung personalities; family, social or school stress; hypoglycemia, and normal pre-pubertal pains.

The main decision your doctor tries to make about stomach pains is whether your child has a condition which, if left untreated, could be harmful. This is a medical dilemma. The doctor doesn't want to do every test in the book just to see what turns up, nor does he or she want to miss any potentially harmful disease. There is a medical axiom that states that "common illnesses have common causes," so your doctor's evaluation of a child's stomach pains usually starts with the basics: a careful medical history, a thorough physical examination, and basic laboratory tests: a blood count, urinalysis, and a urine culture. If these lead your doctor to suspect any serious underlying disease there may be further medical tests.

If your doctor's screening evaluation doesn't come up with anything, you may have to do some detective work. Keep a diary of your child's stomach pains and try to identify what triggers them. Note the time of day when they occur, any associated symptoms, their relation to mealtimes and times of stress, where and when they occur (at home or at school, on weekends or school days), and any other factors you notice that seem to be related. Also note what makes the pains go away. Evaluate your child's environment: is there stress in the home, at school, among friends? This will be very helpful to your doctor in determining the cause and possible treatment of these pains. (Remember that your doctor is trying to determine if the pain should be treated or if it will subside on its own.)

An elimination diet (see page 133) can determine if allergies or food intolerances are the cause of stomach aches.

Encourage your child to eat a healthy snack at mid-morning and mid-afternoon to prevent blood sugar swings. After-school headaches and abdominal pains are particularly common. Ride a school bus home sometime and you may get a few pains, too.

Appendicitis
It's seldom that a day goes by in a busy pediatric office when the doctor does not get a call from a worried parent saying, "I think she has appendicitis." Appendicitis is actually low on the list of causes of abdominal pain. It is good to be cautious about all of your child's pains. This is a natural consequence of loving and caring for your child. If your parental intuition tells you that your child's abdominal pain is more than a little indigestion, call your doctor, especially if this pain seems different from pains she has had before.

The younger the child the more difficult it is to diagnose appendicitis. The pain is usually slightly to the right of the navel or midway between the navel and the groin. The child usually remains very quiet. If you ask her to jump up and down, she either will not do it or after one jump will bend over and pinpoint the pain. The area around the pain is quite tender. When you press it the child will tense her abdomen; when you suddenly remove your hand, she will wince. A low-grade fever, vomiting, and loss of appetite are associated with appendicitis. Fever and chills with abdominal pain should always be reported to your doctor. But if your child is running and jumping and eating well, she does not have appendicitis.

CHAPTER 7

Allergies

The term allergy means altered reaction: something gets into the child's body and causes an unusual reaction. The offending substance, which is called an allergen, may be something in the air, something that touches the skin, or a certain kind of food. These allergens enter the body through the skin, the gastrointestinal tract, or the respiratory tract and stimulate the child's body to produce antibodies. Non-allergic children do not produce antibodies to specific allergens; allergic children do. The presence of the allergen and the antibody in certain tissues, such as the membranes that line the respiratory tract, stimulates the production of substances called histamines. Histamines cause the blood vessels to dilate, which leads to redness of the skin, hives, excessive mucus secretion, runny eyes and nose, a cough, and the accumulation of fluid in the middle ear. Histamines also make the muscles around the breathing passages contract, causing wheezing and asthma.

How can you tell if your child is allergic? The most common signs and symptoms of allergies are:

Runny nose (with clear secretions), watery eyes, seasonal sneezing and wheezing

Chronic cough

Circles under the eyes

Constant sniffling

Frequent colds and/or ear infections

Frequent skin rashes, such as eczema or hives

Night coughs and a stuffy nose in the morning

Coughing during exercise

Diarrhea, abdominal pain, and bloating

Lots of intestinal gas

Fatigue, behavior problems, headaches.

The most common childhood allergic reaction is allergic rhinitis—the stuffy nose, clear watery nasal drainage, itchy eyes, and sneezing typical of hay fever and other inhalant allergies. Because infants and children breathe primarily through their noses, the smallest amount of swelling of the nasal passages can cause a lot of breathing discomfort and produce loud snoring at night. Children with chronic allergic rhinitis have a typical "allergic face": tired and peaked, with an open mouth and dark circles under the eyes ("allergic shiners"). There is a crease across the bridge of the nose caused by rubbing the itchy tip upward with the hand (the "allergic salute"). Most children seem to have a remarkable tolerance for chronic nasal discomfort, making a child's account of how bothered he is somewhat unreliable. I am often amazed at how a child can appear very uncomfortable but complain very little. Children with chronic allergic rhinitis should be taught to blow their noses, rather than sniffing the secretions back inside.

Treating Allergies

Taking care of a child with allergies can prove to be challenging. Try to strike a balance in deciding about treatment of a child's allergies. Children need to live with their allergies. The face of a chronically uncomfortable child brings out feelings of discomfort in the caring parents. Children with chronic allergies often miss many of the fun things of life because of their allergies. They frequently get down in the dumps and wonder "Why am I always sick? Why am I different? Why do I need all these medicines and shots?" Sometimes a cabinet full of medicines and frequent trips to the doctor make a child feel his whole life revolves around his allergies. It is a natural consequence of loving your child that you may tend to overemphasize the illness. Try to help your child understand that he has a medical problem and that most people have problems. You and he together are going to figure out how he can learn to live with it and handle it, and he still will be able to have a lot of fun. Do not think of or refer to this child as "my asthmatic child" or "my allergic child." This is simply your child, who happens to have allergies.

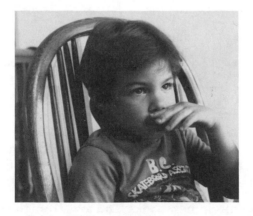

The "allergic salute" is a sign of a runny, itchy nose, the most common symptom of allergy in childhood.

Allergy-Proofing Your Home

If you can determine what things trigger your child's allergic reactions, you can remove many of these things from his environment. Common inhalant allergens include: grass, trees, ragweed pollens, house dust, feathers, mold, mildew, tobacco smoke, wool, animal danders, cooking odors, deodorizers, air fresheners, fireplace smoke, house plants, and aerosols.

Tracking down hidden inhalant allergies begins by "defuzzing" your child's bedroom. Suspect something in the bedroom if your child has a lot of nighttime symptoms or awakens in the morning with a stuffy nose. Try to maintain a dust-free sleeping environment, as much as possible, although it is impossible to remove all the dust from a house. Try the following steps:

Use the bedroom only for sleeping. Dress, study, and play in another room.

Keep the door to the bedroom closed.

Use foam rubber non-allergenic pillows. Avoid feather pillows.

Cover mattress springs with dust-proof covers. Seal the zippers with tape.

Purchase a non-allergenic mattress.

Avoid fuzzy bedding and wash the linens frequently.

Avoid wool blankets and down comforters.

Remove fuzzy stuffed toys from the crib and bed. If your child is highly allergic you may have to put all the fuzzy toys in a garbage bag and temporarily store them in the garage. Synthetic nylon toys stuffed with foam rubber are much less allergenic.

Remove all clothes, books, and toys from the bedroom. Or store clothing in a tightly zippered garment bag.

Move house plants to an area in your home where your child spends little time.

Remove paints such as those used to decorate models.

Look for molds and mildew which collect in damp places. Mold may collect in the bedroom if you use humidifiers or vaporizers frequently.

Clean vaporizers or humidifiers twice weekly to prevent the growth of molds.

During pollen season your child may collect pollen in his hair. Washing his hair nightly before going to bed may minimize any reactions.

If possible, avoid using wall-to-wall carpet in your child's bedroom. Use washable throw rugs on wood or linoleum floors. If this is not possible, get carpet that is less likely to collect dust and vacuum it daily while your child is out of the house. Do not vacuum while your child is in the house. Vacuum cleaners spread tiny dust particles into the air.

Replace dust-collecting drapes or blinds with washable cotton or synthetic curtains or pull-down window shades. Remove upholstered furniture from your child's bedroom. Use wooden chairs or furniture with removable foam cushions and smooth washable covers. Certain kinds of form boards are made with formaldehyde and may be used in the construction of beds. This is a highly allergenic material that should be removed from the bedroom. Any remodeling or redecorating should be done while the child is away—at summer camp, visiting grandma, etc.

Clean and replace air filters frequently, especially with a forced-air heating system. You may need to place accessory filters in the registers in your child's bedroom. Highly allergic children benefit from electronic air filters. (The cost may be covered by your medical insurance.)

Furry or feathered pets should be kept out of your child's bedroom and preferably out of the house. Most children, given the choice, will elect to keep a pet despite allergic symptoms rather than get rid of it. It is wise to be sure that your child is not allergic to an animal before that animal becomes a permanent house guest.

Allergists usually have free booklets on how to create a dust-free environment and still live in it. Most parents find that they do not have to take all of the above steps for their allergic child to improve. It depends on how allergic your child is.

Medications
The medications used to treat allergies are mainly decongestants and antihistamines. These medications are designed to lessen the secretion of mucus and dry up the nose, the sinuses, and the breathing passages. Sometimes it is not wise to use them as this makes the secretions more difficult to cough up and more likely to clog the breathing passages. Antihistamines may cause drowsiness or hyperactivity, personality changes, and sleep difficulties. Children and adults build up tolerance to decongestants and antihistamines, necessitating frequent changes of brand. The goals in treating childhood allergies are to attempt to prevent the secretion of mucus and, if mucus is secreted into the breathing passages, to keep it thin and moving. Stagnant fluid in children, like stagnant water in a pond, often becomes infected, further complicating the allergy.

A new allergy medication called cromolyn (brand names include *Opticrom, Nasalcrom,* and *Intal*) has effects similar to decongestants and antihistamines but does not have the side effects. It is safe for long-term use. Cromolyn is often given as a daily preventive regimen in children with chronic allergies.

Allergy Shots
Allergy shots gradually build up your child's tolerance of an offending allergen so that eventually he will not have an allergic reaction when he comes into contact with it.

There may be specific factors about your child's allergies that may prompt your doctor to recommend allergy shots.

Allergy shots are most effective in three types of allergies: hay fever, asthma, and allergic reactions to bee and wasp stings. They have not been proven to be effective against food allergies and eczema.

Consider how much the allergies bother your child. This is the most important question to ask yourself in deciding how far to go with treatment. Does he miss school, play, or sleep? Is he growing well? Are these allergies a seasonal nuisance that can be easily managed by occasional use of over-the-counter medication, or are they a full-time nuisance that is interfering with your child's growth and development? A child who misses school, who loses sleep, who is not growing and developing well and is in and out of the doctor's office, and who has been on all the usual allergy medications with no signs of improvement is a good candidate for allergy shots. What is the course of the allergies? Is this year worse than last year, or better? Most children will gradually grow out of their allergies. If each month or year seems to be better, then allergy shots are seldom warranted. In deciding whether or not to recommend allergy shots for your child, the doctor considers whether the child will naturally grow out of his hay fever or if there is a risk of the child developing more severe allergies. This risk must be weighed against the discomfort and inconvenience of several years of weekly or twice-weekly injections—with no guarantee that they will work.

Asthma

Parents of a wheezing child often ask, "Is my child asthmatic?" They are usually worried that the child will wheeze all his life long, like Uncle Harry "who has asthma."

Asthma means wheezing. A child may wheeze from an allergy, an infection, or another kind of irritation of the bronchi or breathing passages. The term asthma is usually used to describe long-standing wheezing caused by chronic allergies. It is not correct to label your child asthmatic after a few bouts of wheezing. Wheezing may accompany infectious bronchitis developed during a cold. This is not true asthma. It is only after months or even a year of periodic wheezing caused by allergies that a child should be considered asthmatic.

What happens during an asthmatic attack? The wheezing you hear is caused by air being forced through the child's narrowed breathing passages. During an asthmatic attack the lining of the bronchi reacts to the offending allergen by swelling and pouring out mucus, thus narrowing the air passages. The muscles of the bronchi contract and go into spasm, further narrowing the air passages and obstructing the flow of air. In order to move the amount of air necessary for breathing, the child's chest muscles work harder to push air through these narrowed airways (indrawing of the chest), and he breathes faster. When exhaling, the airways are even narrower, and they produce a wheezing sound. During an asthmatic attack, the child compensates for the difficulty in passing air with three mechanisms: coughing to dislodge the mucus, indrawing of the chest during inhalation to force more air through the bronchi, and forcefully exhaling through narrowed breathing passages, producing a wheezing sound.

Wheezing Worry Signs

Generally, the noisier the wheezing the less there is to worry about. The child must be moving a lot of air in and out to make a lot of noise. Seek medical attention when:

The wheezing child is becoming increasingly exhausted and bothered.

The wheezing becomes less loud, but the indrawing is more noticeable, and the child is breathing more rapidly and seems to be bothered more by the difficulty of getting air. This is called a "tight wheeze" and needs medical attention.

A child who is wheezing noisily but is otherwise himself is of less concern than the silent wheezer. Wheezing during exhalation is of less concern than indrawing during inhalation. Trouble getting air in is of more concern than trouble getting air out.

Chronic cough. A child with a chronic cough may have symptoms similar to asthma. The cough may be the child's only symptom. It is usually worse at night or when the child is exposed to the allergen that sets it off. The allergic reaction causes an outpouring of secretions into the breathing passages. This stimulates coughing as a way of clearing these secretions. The child may not wheeze or have any difficulty breathing: he just has a constant cough. Consult your doctor for treatment.

Exercise asthma. Some children wheeze only during exercise. I have several star athletes in my practice whose exercise asthma is easily controlled by medications taken shortly before participating in a strenuous sport.

Food Allergies

Over the years I have heard just about every medical problem imaginable attributed to food allergies or food intolerance. Food allergy or intolerance produces a variety of signs and symptoms in children. These symptoms may be attributed to other causes; food allergies do masquerade as other problems. Food allergy tends to be either under-diagnosed by the medical profession or over-diagnosed by lay people. Parents are particularly vulnerable to advice about food allergies that may not always be based on reliable sources because love for their children makes them willing to try any suggestion that may put an end to the child's problems. A balanced approach is necessary when parenting the child with possible food allergies.

The most common food allergens are milk and dairy products, chocolate, egg white, shellfish, citrus fruits, tomatoes, yeast, wheat, corn, berries, nuts, peanut butter, pork, and coconut.

Less common allergens include bananas, beef, celery, cherries, chlorinated water, fluoridated water, green peppers, melons, mushrooms, onions, potatoes, prunes, spices, spinach, and synthetic vitamins. Some children cannot tolerate sugar, coffee or other caffeine-containing foods, and artificial food colorings and preservatives, although medically speaking, these reactions may not really be allergies.

Among the foods which seldom cause allergies are apples, apricots, asparagus, barley, beets, carrots, cauliflower, chicken, cranberries, dates, grapes, honey, lamb, lettuce, maple sugar, oats, peaches, pineapples, plums, safflower oil, salmon, soy, squash, sunflower oil, sweet potatoes, tea, and turkey.

These lists are only a general guide. It is possible for any child to be allergic to any food. A child may not react to a small quantity of the food but may have an allergic reaction after injesting large quantities.

Preventing Food Allergies
You can lessen the chances of your child developing food allergies. If you have a strong family history of allergies, the following suggestions may help you prevent the development of allergies in your child:

Breastfeed your infant for at least one year.

Delay introducing solid foods until your infant shows definite signs of readiness for them.

Begin with less allergenic foods (rice, bananas, yellow vegetables) when starting solids.

Avoid giving mixtures of foods to an infant who is less than one year old. If he has an allergic reaction, it will be difficult to tell which food is at fault.

Withhold potentially allergenic foods (see list above) until your child is more than one year old.

How to Track Down Food Allergies

An elimination diet is the key to tracking down your child's food allergies. You eliminate possible allergens and see if the symptoms clear up. Start your elimination diet at a time of the year when other factors will not cloud the detection of food allergies. Do not start a diet at holiday times, near birthdays or other celebrations, or during pollen seasons or home remodeling.

Focus on objective symptoms and signs that you feel may be due to food allergy or intolerance, for example, skin rash, wheezing, runny nose, diarrhea, or abdominal pain. It is hard to be objective about signs such as headaches, behavior changes, hyperactivity, or school problems. Every treatment can have a placebo effect; when you try a new treatment you may see results because you expect to, even if the treatment itself has not really had an objective effect.

Eliminate the most common food allergens first: milk and dairy products, wheat, eggs, nuts, chocolate, corn, and citrus fruits. You may also wish to eliminate colas and other caffeine-containing beverages, sugar, and artificial food colorings and preservatives. Avoid these foods for the first week.

You may be asking, "For heaven sakes, what *can* my child eat?" During this first week your child's diet will consist mainly of meat (except for hot dogs and luncheon meats which may contain artificial coloring), fruits, and vegetables (except for corn). In order to completely eliminate these foods from the diet, you will need to read labels carefully, watching especially for dairy and wheat products. Whey and casein are milk products, and their appearance in the label's list of ingredients makes that food forbidden. Macaroni is made of wheat, noodles may contain eggs, and canned soups may contain both wheat and dairy products. Your child can eat rice crackers and rice bread. (Look for these at the health food store if your supermarket doesn't have them.)

After a week on the elimination diet, you should see some improvement in your child's symptoms. If you don't, you may have to eliminate more foods the next week. Once you have seen some improvement, introduce the eliminated foods back into your child's diet slowly, one food at a time every four days. (This is called a challenge.) If any allergic symptoms reappear, this food is the probable cause, and it goes on your child's list of forbidden foods. If you want to be super-scientific you could eliminate the food for another week and bring it back for a second challenge to see if the same thing happens again. Most parents elect to take only the first challenge.

If your child is not highly allergic and you do not suspect multiple food allergies, you may eliminate one potentially allergenic food at a time, but it may take a lot longer to identify the foods that your child is allergic to.

Some children can tolerate allergenic foods as long as they are not eaten too frequently. These children may be placed on a rotation diet. This means that certain foods are not eaten more than once every two to four days. See the chart for a sample rotation diet.

It may take several weeks or months to track down all of your child's food allergies and pinpoint exactly how much of a certain food your child can eat without a reac-

Sample Rotation Diet

Day One	Day Two	Day Three	Day Four
turkey	lamb	chicken	pork
carrots	one variety of fish	squash	another variety of fish
celery		asparagus	
white potato	broccoli	pears	cabbage
cauliflower	spinach	yams	grapes
apples	lettuce		cherries
	sweet potato		cherries
	pineapple		
	peaches		

tion. For more information about food allergies, elimination diets, and rotation diets, see the following references.

References

Allergies and Your Family by Doris Rapp, M.D. (New York: Sterling Publishing, 1982).

Solving the Puzzle of Your Hard-to-Raise Child by William Crook, M.D. (New York: Random House, 1987). Available from La Leche League International.

CHAPTER 8

Common Infectious Diseases

Many of what used to be common diseases in childhood
are not so common anymore, thanks to the development
of immunizations that protect children against measles,
polio, whooping cough, mumps, diphtheria, and rubella.
Some of these diseases are still around, however, and children who have not been immunized may catch them.
There are other infections for which there are no
immunizations.

Chicken Pox

The day before the chicken pox rash appears the child
may feel entirely well, or she may have mild flu-like symptoms with a low-grade fever. The most striking feature
of the chicken pox rash is how rapidly the spots change.
In the first few hours the rash may appear as a few dot-
ted red areas about the size of a match head. These ini-

tial spots resemble insect bites and first appear on the trunk and face. Within a few hours they change to look like clear blisters on red bases, then cloudy blisters which break and develop a scab. New crops of spots appear all over the trunk, scalp, face, arms, and legs while the older spots are crusting over and healing. Within a few square inches of skin you may see the rash in all four stages.

In the first few hours of chicken pox it is often impossible to tell these spots from other rashes. Parents may think that they are insect bites, and teenagers may decide they have a fresh crop of pimples. Chicken pox is most contagious in the early stage of the rash. If you suspect that your child has chicken pox, keep her away from other children and check on her rash every few hours. If she has chicken pox, the spots will blister within the next several hours and crust over usually within the same day. Bites and pimples won't change much over 24 hours. Bites are most common on the lower legs, the arms, and the hands, whereas chicken pox usually begins on the trunk and face. The chicken pox rash is seldom found on the palms of the hands or the soles of the feet. The spots of chicken pox may also be present in the mouth and in the vagina, which causes intense itching. The lymph glands swell in the region of the spots, especially beneath the scalp along the nape of the neck.

Contagiousness
Chicken pox is one of the most common and most contagious of childhood infectious diseases. It is most common in late winter and early spring. The incubation period (the period of time from exposure to the disease to the time when the rash appears) is between 10 and 20 days with an average of 14 days. Consider your child contagious from a day before the spots first appear to the day they have all crusted over and no new spots appear, usually seven

to ten days after the initial rash. Chicken pox is highly contagious and is spread either by contact with the eruptions (before they scab over) or by droplet spread. The dry scabs (crusts) are not contagious. If one child in the family has chicken pox, there is a 90 percent chance that the other children will also develop the illness. Immunity is usually lifelong; it is rare to have chicken pox a second time. Once you've had it, it is all right to be around a child with chicken pox; you are immune and will not carry the virus. If the mother has had chicken pox, her immunities will protect the newborn from the disease for the first three to six months. This immunity usually wears off by one year.

Chicken pox is a mild disease in children and rarely causes complications. It can be more serious in certain high-risk individuals, and children with chicken pox should stay away from these people to avoid giving them the disease. These include children or adults whose immune systems are not working properly—who are immunocompromised because they are receiving chemotherapy, taking cortisone, or have an underlying immune disease. Because of their depressed immune function, these individuals are particularly susceptible to developing prolonged and complicated cases of chicken pox. Chicken pox is usually more severe in adolescents and adults. Some adults may not recall ever having had chicken pox, but they may have had a mild enough case to have developed immunity even though it was never actually diagnosed as chicken pox.

Children with chicken pox should also be kept away from pregnant women who are not immune. There is a slight risk that the disease may cause damage to the fetus, especially if contracted in the first half of pregnancy. Studies have shown that the risk of fetal defects following chicken pox infection during the first three months of pregnancy is between two and three percent.

What happens if a mother develops chicken pox shortly before delivering her baby? Here are the recommendations of the American Academy of Pediatrics: in mothers who develop chicken pox within five days before or two days after delivery, about half of the infants can be expected to develop chicken pox. These infants should be given an injection of chicken pox immunoglobulin and isolated from other infants for 21 days. It is okay to bring a new baby home from the hospital even if the children at home have chicken pox, as long as the mother has had the disease. If the mother can not recall having chicken pox, it is wise to isolate the new baby from the older children for a period of two weeks. If the mother develops chicken pox while her baby is a newborn, the doctor may decide to give the infant chicken pox immunoglobulin to protect him from the disease.

Vaccines for chicken pox.   If a high-risk individual is exposed to chicken pox, an injection of chicken pox immunoglobulin will usually prevent that person from contracting chicken pox. At present these injections are given only to patients for whom chicken pox may be a serious disease. A chicken pox vaccine is currently being tested for routine use in all children. It will probably be available for general use within a few years.

Treatment of Chicken Pox
Treating chicken pox involves controlling the fever and trying to ease the itching, and keeping your child from scratching. If your child is running a fever, give the appropriate dose of acetaminophen (see page 57). **Do not give aspirin to a child with chicken pox.** The child may go outside in a cool, shady spot.

Itching is the main problem with chicken pox. Try the following anti-itch measures:

> Cut your child's fingernails as short as possible. Tell her not to scratch, and explain that scratching may cause scars and make the chicken pox worse. Have your child wear mittens to bed at night.

Sweating increases itching. Dress your child in light-weight clothes and help her keep cool.

A cool shower or bath three or four times a day is soothing.

Add soothing compounds to the bath water: baking soda (two cupfuls), cornstarch (four tablespoons), or an over-the-counter preparation from your pharmacy (Aveeno Bath, Domeboro). All of these solutions may also be used on a wet washcloth to soak and soothe skin eruptions.

Apply calamine lotion to the itchy scabs and blisters.

Over-the-counter antihistamines may be helpful. If the itching is particularly uncomfortable and keeps the child awake, check with your doctor about a prescription antihistamine.

Some parents have reported that tea is effective in relieving itching from chicken pox in the mouth.

Prevent scarring. While most chicken pox eruptions disappear without a trace in a few months, some may leave scars. Cut fingernails short and strongly discourage scratching, especially on the face. Have the child wear mittens at night so that she can't scratch. In the past few years I have treated many severe cases of chicken pox with a burn cream (Silvadene). This cream prevents superimposed bacterial infections from developing and seems to enhance the healing and prevent scarring, similar to the way it works on burns. Check with your doctor about the use of a burn cream. Avoid sunburn on healing chicken pox areas. Sun damage while the skin is trying to regain its lost pigment can cause permanent discoloration.

Chicken pox is an uncomfortable illness, but not a serious one. Complications such as pneumonia and encephalitis are rare. Sometimes the eruptions may develop a secondary bacterial infection and need treatment with an antibiotic cream.

Measles

Measles is a highly contagious viral infection which is seldom seen anymore because of the measles vaccine. But because not all children have been vaccinated, the disease still occasionally turns up. Measles begins like a common cold with a cough, runny nose, fever, and red, watery eyes which are very sensitive to light. The cough and cold symptoms worsen, and the fever rises to around 104 °F. At the height of the fever, around the fourth or fifth day, a rash appears, beginning on the forehead around the hairline and gradually spreading downward to cover the whole body in the next three days. The rash then begins to fade and disappear, starting again at the forehead and working its way down. On the face and upper body the rash is red and raised and runs together (confluent). On the extremities, the rash may be in distinct patches.

Measles is often confused with other viral illnesses, but it has several distinguishing features. The measles rash appears at the height of the fever, and the fever breaks shortly after the rash appears. Children with measles nearly always have a severe cough. Measles produces white spots on the inside of the cheeks that resemble grains of salt on a red base. These are called Koplik spots. The measles rash is very pronounced, confluent, and deep red, unlike the patchy pinkish-red rashes caused by other viruses. A child with measles appears quite ill, unlike the milder symptoms produced by other viruses.

The incubation period for measles is 8 to 12 days from exposure to the onset of symptoms. The child is contagious from one to two days before the onset of symptoms (three to five days before the rash) to four days after the appearance of the rash.

Treatment of Measles

Treatment for measles consists of rest, fever-lowering medications, lots of fluids, and cough medicines. Because conjunctivitis (red, watery, but not draining, eyes) is nearly always found with measles, the child may be sensitive to bright sunlight, so keep her environment dark. Try to keep your child comfortable until the illness subsides.

Measles usually subsides within seven to ten days without any other treatment. However, complications are more common with measles than with many of the other viruses. These complications include ear infections, pneumonia, and encephalitis. In fact, the main reason for giving the measles vaccine is not to prevent the rash but to avoid the risk of serious complications (mainly encephalitis) that were very common in the days before the vaccine. A severe headache, increasing lethargy and drowsiness, persistent vomiting, and a diminishing level of alertness are worrisome signs in a child with measles; call your doctor if these occur. Children or young adults may occasionally get measles even though they have been given the vaccine. This form of measles is usually mild and uncomplicated.

Measles can be prevented or significantly lessened in a susceptible person by giving measles immunoglobulin within six days of exposure. This protection lasts only a few months and should be followed by immunization with the live measles vaccine.

Mumps

Mumps is a contagious childhood disease caused by a virus which sets up camp in the parotid gland (saliva gland) of the neck. It begins as a vague flu-like illness with fever, nausea, vomiting, headache, and general tiredness. A day later the child may notice pain beneath the earlobe. Usually by the third day of the illness the parotid gland beneath the earlobe becomes obviously swollen and tender. The gland continues to swell on one or both sides giving the child the appearance of "chipmunk" cheeks. The swelling usually subsides by seven to ten days.

The incubation period for mumps is usually from 16 to 18 days, but mumps may occur as early as 12 and as late as 25 days after exposure. The child is considered contagious from one to two days before symptoms appear (around five days before the swollen glands appear) until the glands are no longer swollen or tender. Usually the glands in both sides of the neck are swollen, but in one out of four children swelling is apparent only on one side.

Many children who are exposed to mumps do not develop obvious signs but are infected enough to develop a lasting immunity. It is estimated that 50 percent of adults who think they never had mumps are immune to the disease. Parents may confuse mumps with other types of swollen glands such as those associated with throat infections. These glands are lower and further forward, toward the middle of the jaw bone; the parotid gland is higher, toward the back of the jaw bone and just beneath the earlobe. The swollen glands caused by mumps are exquisitely tender to the touch.

Mumps is usually a mild illness and does not make the child very sick. Although swelling of the parotid glands may be the only sign that you can see, mumps may involve many organs throughout the body, mainly the heart, brain, testicles, and gastrointestinal organs. When mumps involves the vital organs, serious complications such as encephalitis may result. The main reason for encouraging the use of the mumps vaccine is to prevent the complications, not just the swollen glands and a week of missing school.

Treatment for Mumps
Do what you can to keep your child comfortable during mumps. Use fever-lowering medication. (See page 57 for dosages.) Give her soft foods that don't require chewing, such as soup, yogurt, applesauce, and homemade "smoothies," since the swelling may make it painful for her to move her jaw. Call your doctor if the child has a severe headache, is increasingly lethargic or drowsy, is vomiting persistently, or is demonstrating a decreasing level of alertness.

Rubella (German Measles)

Rubella is a virus which makes a child only mildly sick. It begins as a vague, flu-like illness with a low fever (100° to 101°F), general tiredness, and a slight cold. Rubella is usually not suspected until several days later when the rash appears. The rubella rash is mild; it is pinkish-red rather than purple-red like the measles rash. It develops, spreads, and disappears more quickly than the measles rash, usually by the third day. The rubella rash usually appears on the face in distinct patches, whereas the measles rash tends to run together. As with many other viruses, the lymph glands are usually swollen along the hairline at the nape of the neck and behind the ears.

I find that diagnosing rubella can be difficult, since both the symptoms and the rash are very mild and they are like many other viruses. It is estimated that one-quarter to one-half of German measles infections are so mild as to go unrecognized. Rubella is more common among older children and adolescents than among preschoolers. Teenagers with German measles may often experience joint pains.

The incubation period for rubella is from 14 to 21 days. The child may be considered contagious from a few days before to seven days after the appearance of the rash.

Rubella seldom bothers the child. Complications such as encephalitis are rare. The main health concern with rubella is not with children but with pregnant women who are not immune to the virus. Rubella infection during pregnancy can cause fetal abnormalities (rubella syndrome). If you are pregnant and have not had rubella (or are not sure if you did), here are the steps you should take if you have been exposed to a child with German measles during the time that she is contagious:

Your doctor can do a blood test to determine whether you are immune to rubella. (About 85 percent of women of childbearing age have antibodies to rubella and are therefore immune to it.)

If you are not immune, another blood test can detect
if you have been recently infected with rubella. If
this blood test does not show the presence of or a
rise in rubella antibodies, you may have been
exposed to rubella without you or your baby
becoming infected.

If you have been infected with rubella during pregnancy,
there is a risk of giving birth to a baby with rubella syndrome or of having a miscarriage. The chances of these
complications occurring are greater in early pregnancy.
Rubella infection in the second half of pregnancy seldom
harms the baby. Consult your doctor concerning the risks
to your fetus if you have been infected with rubella during pregnancy.

As part of routine medical care, a blood test is performed, either during pregnancy or shortly after birth,
to see if a mother carries antibodies to rubella. If not, it
is wise for the mother to receive the rubella vaccine
shortly after birth. Your doctor may suggest that you wait
a few months after receiving the rubella vaccine before
becoming pregnant, just to be safe.

A child or adult who has just received the rubella vaccine cannot infect others with the virus. Even women who
have received the rubella vaccine early in pregnancy, before they knew they were pregnant, have not produced
babies with rubella syndrome.

Roseola

Roseola is a common viral infection that occurs most often between six and eighteen months of age. It is sometimes called "baby measles," and it may be your baby's
first viral illness and first high fever. Roseola is characterized by the sudden onset of a high temperature (103°
to 105°F) in a previously well child. Parents are usually
surprised that the fever is so high, because the child does
not act very sick. The temperature goes down with the
usual fever-lowering measures, and goes up and down as

they wear off and are repeated. The child seems almost well when the fever drops, but may become quite irritable when the fever rises again. The fever is usually higher at night. This up-and-down pattern continues for about three days. Then the fever drops as suddenly as it began. Within a day after the fever drops, a faint, rose-pink rash appears, first on the trunk and then spreading to the face and upper parts of the extremities. This rash fades if you press on it and is much less intense than the rashes of other illnesses. You may not even notice it. It usually lasts no more than twenty-four hours. Usually there are no other symptoms, although sometimes a child may have some slight cold symptoms and swollen glands on the back of the neck and behind the ears.

Nothing is known about the contagiousness or incubation period of roseola. It is safe to assume that your child is no longer contagious once the fever has disappeared. Treating a child with roseola consists of treating the fever. (See Chapter Four for suggestions.)

The problem with roseola is not the disease, but the diagnosis. Because the rash does not appear until the fever is gone and the child is better, you or the doctor may suspect that an infant with a fever has roseola, but the diagnosis cannot be confirmed until a few days later. Typically, when a child is brought to the doctor's office for suspected roseola, all that can be said for certain is that the child has a fever of unknown origin. The doctor examines the child and finds no apparent cause for the fever. The eardrums may appear red, but they usually do with a fever. The child doesn't seem sick, and the fever is easily controlled with medication. The doctor concludes that this is probably roseola. No antibiotic is necessary, and the only treatment is to keep the fever under control. Remember the important part of your doctor's advice: "If she gets sicker, call me." Roseola does not get worse; it just may not get better for a few days. After the fever breaks and the rash appears, the suspected diagnosis is confirmed.

Sometimes an infant with a fever of unknown origin is given an antibiotic because the doctor suspects that the child has a bacterial infection. The fever goes down and a rash appears. This can create a diagnostic dilemma. Did the child have a bacterial infection which responded to the antibiotic, causing the fever to go down? Did the child have roseola? Or is the rash an allergic reaction to the antibiotic? Actually, there are noticeable differences between the rash of roseola and those caused by allergies to antibiotics. The roseola rash is short-lasting, faint, non-raised, and pinkish-red. A rash caused by an allergic reaction to an antibiotic is usually all over the body, lasts three or four days, is red, raised, and itchy, and looks worse than the roseola rash. Nevertheless, I suspect that many children who have been labeled allergic to penicillin actually had roseola in infancy.

Influenza

There are many types of influenza viruses. The flu generally occurs during the winter months and is characterized by some or all of the following symptoms: fever, generalized aches and pains (muscle aches, headaches, abdominal pains), vomiting, diarrhea, cough, runny nose, fatigue, paleness, loss of appetite, and photophobia (high sensitivity to sunlight). Flu tends to occur in epidemics. Other family members, schoolmates, and friends may be affected with similar signs and symptoms. Like most viruses the incubation period averages around fourteen days, and the child is contagious from the day before the onset of symptoms until the time the fever and most of the severe symptoms are gone. It is common for the child to remain tired for a week or two following the flu, but during this time she is not contagious. Treatment consists of fever control (pages 56-60), prevention of dehydration (pages 109-112), and comforting measures (Chapter Two).

Is It Really Flu?
One of the main problems with the flu is that there is often more going on than "just the flu." Many other illnesses are missed during flu epidemics, because of the tendency to believe that a sick child has whatever "bug" all the other children seem to have at that time. I have seen many children whose symptoms sounded like flu over the phone but who, on examination, actually had other problems which may mimic the flu: pneumonia, sinus infections, urinary tract infections, and, most serious, meningitis. (See page 150 for a discussion of meningitis.)

Consider the following in deciding whether or not to consult your doctor about what seems to be a case of flu:

Flu does not get worse rapidly from day to day.

With flu, children cannot usually point to the site of pain the way they can with an earache or sore throat. The aches and pains of the flu are more generalized.

With flu, the fever goes up and down, is worse at night, and is easily lowered a couple of degrees by fever-lowering medications, though it may go back up again.

A persistently high fever unresponsive to fever-lowering measures is seldom caused by the flu.

Persistent vomiting and increasing drowsiness are more than just the flu.

Signs of dehydration are more than just the flu.

If your child has a persistently high fever, localized pain, persistent vomiting, increasing lethargy, or signs of dehydration, consult your doctor, even if you think it's nothing more than flu. If your child seems to be getting worse during a suspected flu illness, consult your doctor.

Post-flu complications.   Since the flu is a virus it usually goes away within a week and is not helped by antibiotics. Sometimes fluid remains in various cavities (sinuses, ears, and chest) after the flu. This fluid attracts bacteria, and a bacterial infection may commence as the flu is subsiding. This is more than the flu lingering on; bacterial infections need medical treatment with antibiotics. If your child's flu is not going away, watch for signs of ear, sinus, or bronchial infections.

Meningitis

Meningitis is one of the most serious infectious diseases. It may be caused by either a virus or bacteria. Viral meningitis is usually much less serious than bacterial meningitis. Meningitis is an infection and inflammation of the meninges, the membranes covering the brain and spinal cord. The germs causing meningitis may enter the body just like a cold. In fact, meningitis often begins as a cold, sore throat, ear infection, or other common infection of childhood. The germ travels into the meninges via the bloodstream. The younger the infant or child, the more difficult it is to diagnose meningitis. The following signs and symptoms should alert parents to the possibility of meningitis:

The child is increasingly ill with a persistent medium to high fever, rapid heartbeat, chills, pallor.

There is increasing lethargy and drowsiness, and a decreasing level of alertness. (These are signs of neurological involvement.)

The child has difficulty walking and is unwilling to stand up.

There are signs of neck and spinal column pain or stiffness. It hurts to move. The child may want to lie very still. She is unable or unwilling to bend her neck to touch her chin to her chest.

The child has persistent vomiting and/or headache.

If any of the above signs and symptoms occur, seek medical attention immediately. Neck stiffness in particular may be difficult for parents to evaluate themselves, so it is important to consult a doctor. There is a condition called **meningism** in which, during a high fever, the child seems unwilling to flex her neck. With meningism, when the fever goes down, the neck stiffness disappears; in meningitis, it doesn't. (There is cause for concern in any illness if a child does not improve significantly when the fever is brought down.)

Meningitis can usually be successfully treated with large doses of intravenous antibiotics for seven to ten days. Depending on how early the diagnosis is made, children often make a complete recovery. This is why it is so important for parents to seek medical attention at the slightest hint of meningitis symptoms. The earlier the diagnosis is made and proper treatment instituted, the more likely that your child will make a complete recovery.

Pinworms

Pinworms are not harmful, but they can be irritating. A pinworm infection often bothers parents more than the child. Pinworms resemble tiny pieces of white thread about one-third of an inch long. Pinworms reside and mate in the child's intestines. The pregnant female then travels down the intestines and out the rectum to lay her eggs around the anal opening, usually at night. All this activity results in intense itching, causing the child to scratch the egg-infested area around her anus and buttocks. These eggs are then picked up on the fingers and beneath the fingernails and are transmitted to the child's mouth, to other children, or to other members of the household. The swallowed eggs hatch in the intestines, mature, mate, and repeat the life cycle.

Pinworm infection is very common. It is estimated that approximately ten percent of the population is infected with pinworms, mainly preschool and school-age children. Parents of infected children also carry the worms. In girls, pinworms may also be found in the vagina, causing intense itching. The female worms usually die after depositing the eggs, so the worms themselves are not transmitted from person to person. The infection is spread only by transferring the eggs. Pinworm eggs can be transmitted only from person to person; they can't be transferred from a person to a thing and then to another person.

Although these tiny parasites have been blamed for every imaginable symptom from appendicitis to learning disabilities, probably the only symptom they can truly be found guilty of is intense itching around the anus, buttocks, or vagina. Pinworms, therefore, constitute more of a nuisance than a real medical problem.

Looking for Pinworms
Suspect pinworms if your child has been waking or is restless at night and is scratching around the anus or vagina, mostly at night. Sometimes the child can be seen squirming while sitting as a way of scratching her bottom. You may actually be able to see pinworms, if you look for them. At night, in the dark, hold your child's buttocks apart and shine a light on the rectum. You may see tiny, thread-like worms. But more often than not, even though you suspect the worms are there, you cannot see them. You can easily capture the eggs by placing the sticky side of a piece of tape (mount it on a popsicle stick or tongue depressor) around the anus in the area of the itch; this test is best performed when your child awakens, before she takes a bath or has a bowel movement. Take the tape to your doctor or to a laboratory where it can be examined under a microscope for pinworm eggs.

Getting Rid of Pinworms
Treatment of pinworms is safe and simple. The child is given a single dose of a prescription medication. The pinworm medication contains a red dye which colors the stool bright red. Since vomiting occasionally occurs shortly after swallowing this medication, it is best administered in a

place where red spills or spit-up will not stain anything. Recurrences are common and can be minimized by treating the whole family and other close contacts of the child all at once and by repeating the initial dosage ten days to two weeks later.

Head Lice

When your child is sent home from school with a note informing you that she has head lice, your first reaction may be embarrassment or even outrage. But having head lice is not a reflection on your housekeeping, your cleaning habits, or your socioeconomic status. Head lice honor even the best of homes with their presence.

The head louse is a tiny parasite, too small to be seen with the naked eye, which punctures the skin of the scalp to feed and deposit its excretory products. This causes intense itching, which is usually the only symptom of lice. Sometimes a secondary bacterial infection may develop, resulting in impetigo-like rashes and tiny boils throughout the scalp. The head louse deposits its eggs (nits) on the base of the hair shaft where they can be seen as tiny, gray, oval-shaped specks firmly cemented to the hair. Nits are clearly visible. After about one week, when the eggs hatch, the mature lice can be transferred from one person to another by sharing clothing or combs and brushes.

To check your child for head lice, examine the hair at the base of the hairline on the back of the child's head or around the ears. Look for nits or evidence of scratching. Nits look different from dandruff. Dandruff is flat and flaky and easily slides up and down on the hair shaft. Nits are oblong and oval and firmly cemented to the hair shaft. Sometimes the lymph glands may be swollen and can be felt at the base of your child's skull.

If you see the nits and suspect that your child has head lice, don't panic. Take action: become a nitpicker! Try an over-the-counter lice shampoo (A200, Rid), following the directions on the package. Using a special fine-toothed comb (which comes in the package of the lice medicine) comb the nits out of the hair. If the over-the-counter shampoo is not effective, obtain a prescription for a lice shampoo from your doctor. This shampoo is potentially more toxic than the over-the-counter shampoos and must be used carefully, following your doctor's directions exactly. It is normal for the itching to remain for a week or two after the lice and nits have been killed. It is not necessary to use the prescription shampoo repeatedly until the symptoms disappear.

Thoroughly wash personal articles such as combs, brushes, scarves, hats, and bed clothing—anything which touches the hair—in very hot water. Dry clothing and linens in the hot cycle in the dryer. Or have the items dry cleaned. If this is impractical, placing items in a sealed plastic bag for ten days will kill the lice and eggs.

When you spot lice on your child's head, it is not necessary to get rid of the dog or fumigate the house. Lice can be caught only from an infected person or from that person's intimate head apparel. Lice are not transmitted by pets. The most common means of transmission is sharing hats, combs, or brushes. It is not necessary to keep your child home from school if your child has head lice, but tell her not to share combs, brushes, and hats. Often, if one family member has head lice, it is wise to treat the whole family. Parents' reactions to head lice are often worse than the infection itself. It is best not to make a big deal about it. Treat it with a little humor, some nit-picking (literally), and a thorough shampoo. Then send your child back to school.

CHAPTER 9

Common Skin Problems

Skin diseases are particularly distressing to parents and children because they are so readily visible. Skin problems are one of the most common childhood ailments, but they are also the easiest to recognize and treat. This chapter discusses some of the most common skin problems in children as well as what parents need to know to care for their child's skin.

In infants and young children, the outer layer of skin (the epidermis) is thinner than in adults; it gradually thickens as the child matures. The thinner skin plus the child's relatively immature immune system make him more susceptible to skin irritation and infection. The sebaceous glands which produce oil that lubricates the skin are less active in the infant and young child, so the skin becomes dried and chapped more easily, and it is also more susceptible to fungus infections. Infants and children sweat much less than older children and adults, which further contributes to dry skin. During adolescence and early adulthood the skin becomes thicker, the sebaceous glands secrete more lubrication, and the tendency toward dry and easily irritated skin lessens with increasing growth. The thin skin of infants and young children absorbs medications more easily, thus increasing the risk of system-wide side effects from ointments and creams used to treat skin problems.

Taking Care of Skin

There are many kinds of creams, ointments, dressings, and homemade concoctions that can be used to soothe and help heal skin problems. Some, but not all, are helpful.

Baths

Baths are helpful in soothing and cleaning the skin. Twenty minutes in a slightly warm (tepid) bath is particularly soothing. For itchy skin add one or two packets of *Aveeno* (an oatmeal preparation) or one cup of baking soda to the bath water. For dry, scaly skin, add lubricating substances containing mineral oil or lanolin. Avoid products that contain lanolin if your child is allergic to wool.

Soaps. Most mothers seem to have a bit of the mother cat instinct: they love to wash their babies. Most soaps are drying to the skin. Since baby's skin is very susceptible to drying anyway, soaps often aggravate this problem. Use a mild soap *(Neutrogena, Dove)* and avoid excessive scrubbing except in particularly dirty areas such as elbows and knees. The scalp in particular is very susceptible to the over-use of soaps and shampoos. In most babies, a scalp wash once a week and a bath twice a week is plenty, except for daily washing of face and diaper areas. It is best to blot a baby's skin dry rather than to rub it, which may remove natural skin oils. When washing off an infected or injured area, such as a burn, it is better to place the infected area under a stream of water from the faucet than to rub with a wash cloth. Running water is a very effective way to remove germs, dead skin, and debris from infected skin.

Powders, Ointments, Creams, and Lotions

Gone are the days when a baby was sprinkled with perfumed talcum after every bath. (At least I hope those days are gone.) I generally discourage the use of any powders in the care of baby's skin. Talcum powers may be inhaled as they are dusted on, and they may be irritating to the lungs. Perfumed powders mask the natural scent of a baby which, in breastfed babies, is usually very pleasant. When applied in skin creases, such as the groin and neck folds, powders tend to cake. Products containing cornstarch should be particularly avoided on baby's skin since they promote the growth of fungi.

Unless advised by your doctor, it is generally unnecessary to apply oils or lotions to a baby's skin. A baby's skin usually has enough natural oils. Oils and lotions may also promote the growth of skin bacteria. Lubricating solutions (lanolin, mineral oil) may be used on patchy areas of dry skin.

Creams and ointments. When standing at the medicine counter in your pharmacy you will notice the wide variety of topical (meaning applied-to-the-skin) solutions using the term cream or ointment. They are different types of substances and have different uses. Creams are water-based agents which are applied to oozing, blistery, wet eruptions in which the desired effect is to dry up the skin problem. Ointments are petroleum-based compounds which are applied to dry plaque-like skin problems to help soften them.

Compresses

Compresses are wet dressings which soothe itchy and in-flamed skin, dry oozing eruptions, and soften crusts and scales. Two common childhood skin problems which benefit from wet compresses are poison ivy and chicken pox. To make wet compresses use a folded clean cloth such as a diaper, handkerchief, part of an old sheet, or a dish towel. Soak the dressing in a soothing solution (*Domeboro,* one packet to a pint of water). Apply the wet dressing to the skin area for five to ten minutes. As the dressing begins to dry, remove it, and rinse off the infected skin area under cool water from the faucet. Then repeat the compress. Discard the compress after use.

Band-Aids

Band-aids are the panacea for many little hurts of infants and children. But does covering a wound really help it heal? Band-aids are usually more of a psychological boon

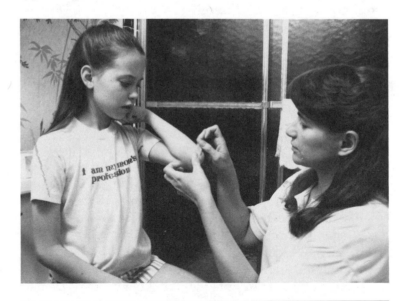

Band-aids help wounds heal—and children like them!

to children. When a little child sees his skin violated by a little "ouchy," band-aids provide great emotional support—a patch for the leak in the body and a trophy for surviving the hurt. A childless person when confronted with a bleeding child with a tiny puncture wound who asks for a band-aid might argue, "Oh, that little cut doesn't need a band-aid." An experienced parent won't bother with reasoning; he or she will quickly apply the comforting band-aid.

Whether to leave a wound open and let it breathe or to cover it has been debated for centuries. Current research suggests that wounds heal better in a moist, occlusive environment which prevents germs from entering the wound and the wound from drying out. Specialists now believe that letting a scab form and drying out a wound do not promote healing as much as covering the wound and keeping it moist.

Eczema

Eczema is a patchy, scaly, intensely itchy skin condition which is either inherited as a family skin problem or is caused by allergy (usually a food or contact allergy). Eczema usually occurs in square-inch-size patches on the cheeks, on the arms, inside the elbows, and behind the knees. Itching is the hallmark of eczema, and scratching only causes more irritation which in turn causes more itching. Over time, the itch-scratch cycle produces thickened skin. Sometimes the scratching breaks down the protective layer of outer skin and allows a superimposed bacterial infection to develop.

Treatment of Eczema
Try to figure out if the eczema is caused by allergy. The most common eczema-producing allergens are soaps, detergents, fabrics (especially wool), foods (eggs, dairy, and wheat), and carpets. Stress may also precipitate eczema, so any measures that will make the environment less

Common Skin Medications

Topical antibiotic creams and ointments *(Polysporin, Neosporin, Bacitracin, Bactroban*)*	Antibacterial applied to abrasions, scratches, oozing and infected skin conditions—any skin condition in which the outer layer of skin is damaged, allowing entry of bacteria.
Calamine lotion	Dries, cools, and soothes inflamed skin.
Domeboro, tablets or packets	Soothes and dries oozing, blistered, and itchy skin conditions such as poison ivy or chicken pox.
Aveeno	Add to bath. Soothes dry, itchy, inflamed skin as in eczema or hives.
Hydrogen peroxide	Used to remove scabs, crust, and dead tissue.
Antifungal medications *(Mycostatin*, Lotrimin*)*	Treatment of fungal infections, mainly of the diaper area.
Cleansing soaps *(Phisoderm, Neutrogena, Cetaphil)*	For cleansing dirty skin; avoid overuse on dry skin.
Emollients *(Keri Lotion, Eucerin, mineral oil)*	For soothing and moisturizing dry, flaky skin.
Zinc oxide cream	Barrier cream for prevention of diaper rash.
Antiseptic solutions *(Hibiclens, Betadine)*	Cleansing infected or potentially infected skin.
Baking soda	When added to bath, soothes itchy skin.
Cortisone creams	Relieves itching, swelling caused by allergic reactions; use only as directed by a physician. Overuse may thin and discolor skin.

* Available by prescription only.

stressful should help relieve eczema. To relieve the itching, try the following:

A cool, humid environment will help lessen problems with eczema. Use a vaporizer or humidifier in your home. The dry air of central heating aggravates eczema. (A week in Hawaii is a great, though expensive, way to relieve chronic and severe eczema)

Avoid excessive use of soap, which is drying to the skin. If soap is necessary, use a creamy, emollient type of soap *(Neutrogena, Dove, Cetaphil Lotion)*.

Emollients such as mineral oil and *Keri Lotion* or lubricating lotions such as *Lubriderm, Eucerin, Nivea* or *Oilated Aveeno* can be used to help soften the skin. (*Keri Lotion* should not be used in children allergic to wool.)

Cut fingernails short to minimize scratching.

If eczema is severe, use wet compresses containing soothing solutions such as *Domeboro.*

Cool non-soapy baths may reduce the itching. Add *Aveeno,* one cup to a tub of tepid water.

Cortisone creams are very effective in the treatment of chronic eczema but should be used only as directed by a physician, only when the eczema is severe and not helped by the above measures, and only in the strength and for the duration of time prescribed by the physician.

Contact Dermatitis

Contact dermatitis produces a rash similar to eczema. It usually does not have a hereditary basis. It is caused by contact with an irritant. The most common skin irritants are new clothing, detergents, and plants such as poison ivy and poison oak. Contact dermatitis due to detergents or clothing is characterized by a pink, raised, scaly, itchy rash over the areas covered by clothing. Sometimes only a part of the clothing, such as the elastic bands on water-proof pants or the plastic lining of disposable diapers is responsible for contact dermatitis, and the rash will appear only in areas in contact with these parts. Treatment of contact dermatitis consists of detecting and removing the offending allergen, cutting the child's fingernails, and, if severe, using all the soothing ideas listed under eczema.

Poison ivy and poison oak. The most uncomfortable types of contact dermatitis come from run-ins with poison ivy or poison oak. The rash is scaly, blistery, raised, and intensely itchy. It often appears in a line where the allergenic leaf has brushed against the skin. The allergic reaction is caused by the oil in the plant. The rash is usually the result of touching the plant, but exposure to oils carried by pollen or by smoke when the plants are burned may also provoke a reaction.

Treatment of poison ivy is directed at slowing down the inflammation, relieving the intense itching, and preventing superimposed infections:

Thoroughly wash your child's skin as soon as possible.

Cool compresses of *Domeboro* solution or a cool bath with *Aveeno* may be soothing.

Sometimes a hot bath will, surprisingly, bring relief from itching. Sometimes a hot bath will temporarily increase the itching, but the itching will subside remarkably after the hot bath is finished.

Calamine lotion may provide some relief.

Cortisone creams, prescribed by your doctor, are especially helpful in providing immediate relief and slowing down the inflammation and itching. In severe cases of poison ivy or poison oak, three days of cortisone tablets may be needed.

A sedative, prescribed by your doctor, may help your child sleep and relieve the itching.

Poison ivy is rarely contagious. Once the oils have been absorbed in the skin or removed by washing, the skin lesions cannot transfer the rash to another person or to other areas of the body.

Hives

Hives, also called urticaria, is an allergic skin reaction that can be recognized by the characteristic wheals: circular, red areas the size of a dime or quarter which have raised, red borders and pale centers. These wheals fade when they are pressed. They spread rapidly and often cover the child's whole body. Hives look worse than they really are. Sometimes they develop a bluish discoloration and resemble bruises. Because of the itching, the child is generally uncomfortable with hives and unable to sleep comfortably. Hives usually disappear within three to four days. Unlike contact dermatitis, hives are an allergic reaction to an allergen which has entered the blood stream, either a food, a drug, venom from an insect bite, or an inhalant allergen. The most common causes of hives include pollens, insect bites, drugs, and foods, especially dairy products, wheat, chocolate, pork, eggs, shellfish, berries, tomatoes, and nuts. Most hives are mild, but sometimes the allergic reaction is severe and the eyelids and hands may be swollen. Swelling of the airways may occur, causing a wheeze or croupy cough.

Treating Hives

If hives are severe and accompanied by swelling of the hands, eyelids, or respiratory passages, your doctor or hospital may need to administer a shot of adrenalin, which usually gives relief in minutes. In less severe cases, try a cool bath with soothing compounds added to the water (Aveeno, Domeboro) or antihistamines taken three or four times a day for several days. Try to figure out what caused the hives. Make a list of foods and other allergens to which your child was exposed in the twenty-four hours before the hives appeared.

Bacterial Infections of the Skin

Impetigo

Impetigo is a bacterial infection of the skin which begins as tiny red spots (resembling picked-at pimples) that become blisters which rupture and produce an oozing, sticky, honey-colored crust. The spots are circular and may be as small as a dime or as large as a quarter. They tend to occur in distinct patches beneath the nose or on the buttocks and arms. Impetigo is particularly common around the entrance to the nose, where the skin around the nostrils appears raw and reddened with a yellow crust.

Impetigo may or may not itch. Scratching spreads the eruptions. Mild impetigo is often caused by streptococcus bacteria. Severe and blistery impetigo is often caused by staphylococcus. The bacteria may invade any area where the top protective layer of skin is broken down by an injury, such as a bite or an abrasion. Picking the skin around the nose or picking a pimple is an invitation for bacteria to come in and set up an infection. It is important for parents to be aware that impetigo, like head lice, is not a reflection of sloppy housekeeping or poor hygiene. Nor is impetigo as contagious as it is sometimes made out to be. You do not have to treat your child like a leper if he has impetigo. It can be transmitted by touching the eruptions, so it is important to tell your child not to touch the rash. Although it is common to find impetigo in several family members at once, it is rarely necessary to keep the child with impetigo out of school.

Treating impetigo. Impetigo is usually treated with antibiotics, either applied directly to the rash (topical) or given orally (systemic). Consult your doctor for advice. A prescription antibacterial cream *(Bactroban)* is particularly effective in mild to moderate cases of impetigo. Systemic antibiotics (usually penicillin) are usually prescribed in moderate to severe cases. Until the recent advent of improved topical antibacterial creams, systemic antibiotics were routinely used to treat impetigo. In severe cases of impetigo caused by staphylococcus, a broad spectrum antibiotic may be used. Here are some other suggestions:

If possible, cover the lesions with an antibacterial ointment and a dressing that will keep air out and moisture in. This speeds healing and minimizes spread to other parts of your child's body and to other individuals.

Cut your child's fingernails and tell him not to scratch or touch the lesions.

Wet compresses made with a solution of *Domeboro* may be used to relieve the itching.

It is necessary to correctly diagnose and treat impetigo. Although most cases of impetigo are limited to a nasty-looking skin eruption, the bacteria may enter the blood stream and cause infection in other organs, such as inflammation of the kidneys.

Cellulitis
Cellulitis is a bacterial infection of the tissues underneath the skin. It is characterized by the four signs of skin infection: redness, swelling, tenderness, and warmth. Like impetigo, cellulitis usually begins with an injury to the superficial layer of the skin (abrasions, puncture wounds) that provides an entry point for bacteria. These bacteria spread rapidly through the tissues under the skin and produce cellulitis. The affected area, usually an extremity, is very swollen, hot, and tender. Lymph glands in the area are swollen and tender. The child usually has a fever and is generally unwell. One of the earliest signs of cellulitis is red streaks on the skin extending from the area of superficial infection. Treatment is always with antibiotics. If severe, hospitalization and intravenous antibiotics may be necessary.

Boils

Boils are bacterial skin infections. They resemble pimples which have gotten out of control and are severely infected. They may be as small as a pea or as large as a marble.

A boil shows the four signs of infection: redness, swelling, tenderness, and warmth. Boils begin when bacteria penetrate the skin and proliferate within a small area. For example, bacteria may enter the skin at the base of a hair and begin multiplying in the nearby sebaceous gland. This pocket of pus gradually forms a wall around itself, and although it may cease growing, it does not disappear. Boils often occur around hair shafts or in areas under pressure, such as the buttocks. In older children and adolescents, a boil may be the result of an infected pimple or infected acne.

Treating boils. Since a boil is really pus under pressure, home treatment is aimed at draining the pus from the boil. First, apply moist heat (a wash cloth with hot water) for several minutes at least six times a day. Continue these hot compresses until the skin at the head of the boil becomes very thin or "ripe" (this is called "bringing the boil to a head") and a day or so later, ruptures and drains. Continue the application of moist heat for several days after the drainage begins in order to clear all of the infected pus from the boil and keep the draining center of the boil open. Do not squeeze the boil as this may break down the natural wall around the boil and cause the infection to spread into nearby tissues, resulting in cellulitis. Cover the boil with a topical antibiotic cream and an occlusive bandage (one that will keep air out and moisture in). If, after you think you have gotten out all the pus, the child still feels pain when pressure is applied to the boil, it may be that the "core" of the boil has not been removed. Your doctor may need to open the boil further and remove the rest of the pus. If the boil does not seem to be going away with this home treatment or if it does not become ripe and drain on its own, consult your doctor. He or she may decide to cut and drain the boil in the office or at the hospital. This is called lancing the boil. Systemic antibiotics may also be necessary.

Scabies

Scabies (from the Latin scabere, to scratch) is a skin irritation caused by a mite the size of a pinpoint. It is moderately contagious, being transmitted from person to person or from contact with intimate apparel and bedding. The mite attaches itself to the skin, usually in moist skin folds such as between the fingers and toes, under the arms, or inside the elbows. It burrows under the skin where it lays its eggs. The mites themselves and the eggs hatching under the skin produce intense itching, especially at night. Initially, the rash of scabies may resemble tiny flea bites, chicken pox, eczema, impetigo, or a combination of all of these rashes. But the unique feature of scabies is the inch-long tiny burrows which can be seen on the surface of the skin. The diagnosis of scabies is often difficult because the scratching it provokes produces another rash on top of the scabies rash. Scabies is often suspected when an itchy rash that has been present for several weeks is not getting better with simple home remedies and seems to be spreading. Sometimes the only way to diagnose scabies is for your doctor to scrape the tunnel area of the skin and use a microscope to look for the mite in the scrapings.

Treating Scabies
The main treatment for scabies is a special lotion prescribed by your doctor. This is best applied at night, right after a warm bath during which you have scrubbed the lesions with a stiff brush to allow the lotion to penetrate better. It is common for the itching to persist even after the mites have been killed by one or two applications of the lotion. Avoid the temptation to keep applying the lotion until the itching has disappeared. Over-use of these prescription lotions may be harmful. Cool baths with *Aveeno*, cool compresses of *Domeboro* solution, or

calamine lotion can be used to soothe the itch. Launder intimate clothing and bedding. You do not have to scrub down the whole house because mites die within a few hours if they don't find a warm body to nest on.

Ringworm

Ringworm is not caused by a worm. It is a fungus infection of the skin or scalp that is characterized by a ring-like rash. The rash begins as a small, round, red area on the skin. The center of the rash clears, leaving an elevated, red, scaly ring with a pale center. Ringworm is mildly contagious and is spread by contact or by scratching; it is not as contagious as impetigo. The child with ringworm need not be isolated. Ringworm may itch, but usually not intensely. It is most common on the face and scalp, and the rash usually varies in size from a dime to a quarter.

Over-the-counter anti-fungal medications, such as *Tinactin* or *Micatin,* applied three times a day are usually effective against ringworm. Be prepared for the rash to take several weeks to disappear. It is common for the skin to be whitish temporarily after the rash disappears. If after several weeks of home treatment, the ringworm is still there, see your doctor for confirmation of the diagnosis and possibly, a prescription cream.

Sunburn

Infants and children are particularly prone to sunburn. The younger the infant, the more sensitive the skin is to sun, and naturally, fair skin is more sensitive to sunburn than dark skin. Some exposure to sun is necessary, as sunlight is a valuable source of vitamin D for your child. To prevent sunburn:

> Keep infants and children out of the intense spring and summer sun, especially between 11:00 AM and 3:00 PM.

If your child is fair-skinned (blond or red hair and light-color eyes mean fair skin), schedule outside play for early to mid-morning or late afternoon.

Cover your child with a bonnet or baseball hat, a long-sleeved shirt, and long pants.

Beware of reflected sunlight. Sunlight reflects upward from sand and water. Sitting in the shade or under an umbrella does not guarantee protection from reflected light.

Using sunscreens for infants and children. Sunscreens protect the skin from damaging rays of the sun, but the same elements which protect your child's skin may also be harmful. There is some experimental evidence that the compound PABA, found in many sunscreens, may be

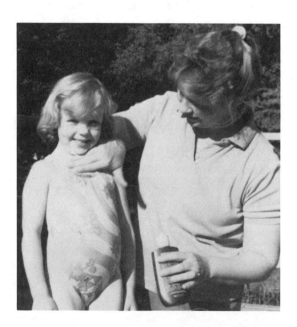

Sunscreens should be reapplied every hour if children are swimming or playing in the water.

harmful to children. Until more is known, it is safest to use a sunscreen that does not contain PABA. Choose one with a sun protection factor (SPF) of 15 or higher.

It's a good idea to make certain that your child is not allergic to a particular sunscreen. Apply a small amount of it on the underside of the forearm and watch for a reaction. (Do this a few days *before* the big trip to the beach.) If a raised, red, itchy rash soon appears, your child may be allergic to this particular product, and you will need to try another one.

Apply sunscreen liberally to all exposed areas of the skin, especially the cheeks and forearms. Do this at least fifteen minutes before going outside to allow the protective ingredients to sink in. Avoid using sunscreen close to the eyes, as children tend to rub their eyes and some products may be irritating. Reapply liberally about every hour. If your child will be in the water, look for a waterproof sunscreen and reapply every hour.

What to do about sunburn.   Most sunburns are first-degree burns; the skin is reddened but not blistered. If the skin is blistered (a second-degree burn) or your child is running a fever, consult your doctor. Cool compresses and cool soothing baths with *Aveeno* or baking soda added to the water may help soothe sunburned skin.

CHAPTER 10

Child Safety and Accident Prevention

One out of three childhood deaths is caused by an accident. It's important for parents to know why children are prone to accidents and what sorts of accidents can happen, as well as how to prevent them.

The Accident-Prone Child

Around the time their child is one year of age most parents will discover if she is accident-prone. How a child learns to walk will often give you clues about how impulsive and accident-prone she is. Some children slowly but steadily go through the developmental progression of sitting, crawling, pulling up to a stand, walking while holding on to furniture, and finally walking alone. This type of child is aware of her own developmental skills at each stage and will not rush forward into a new skill until she has comfortably mastered the previous one. The impulsive child, on the other hand, will often go through this

Accidents that Occur at Different Developmental Stages

Knowing what kinds of accidents to watch for at a given age
and stage may help you to prevent them.
Birth to six months
   Falls—rolling off changing tables or out of infant seats
   Crib accidents
   Burns from bath water
   Auto accidents
Six months to twelve months (crawling to walking)
   Toy accidents from sharp edges, strings, small mouth-
   able parts
   Grabbing accidents: burns from hot coffee, cuts from
   breakables
   High chair accidents
   Falls against sharp table corners
   Electric burns from sockets and cords
   Cigarette burns
   Walker and stroller accidents
   Auto accidents
One year to two years (walking and exploring)
   Exploring accidents in storage cupboards, medicine
   cabinets
   Climbing accidents on stairs and furniture
   Eating poisonous plants
   Cuts
   Unguarded water hazards (pools, ponds, and bath
   tubs)
   Auto accidents
Preschool and school age
   Playground accidents
   Fire accidents: matches, lighters
   Yard and street accidents
   Tricycle and bicycle accidents
   Kidnappings
   Auto accidents
Teens
   Sports accidents
   Drug and alcohol abuse
   Moped accidents
   Auto accidents

developmental progression quickly, walk early (before eleven months), and dart unexpectedly from one piece of furniture to another. She doesn't seem to mind stumbling frequently in her relentless pursuit of a specific goal or in her sheer enjoyment of motion. Impulsive, very active, very busy children are often the ones who are the most accident-prone. For most babies and toddlers, the desire to perform a new skill develops before they are able to accomplish it safely, but less impulsive children are more calculating and do not try a new task until they can comfortably handle it. Impulsive children often do not think before they act and may try to do things before they are ready.

Watch for "mouthers." While some infants seem to know intuitively which objects should not be put in the mouth, other infants and children seem to have an insatiable need to put any small mouthable object into their mouths. Watch your child play with small objects. The child who picks up a small object and studies it before testing it in her mouth is less likely to swallow dangerous objects than the child whose first impulse with any new object is to put it in her mouth.

Beware of the "darter." Some children frequently and impulsively dart away from a parent. They do not seem to need the security of frequent checks with home base. The so-called independent child may be more accident-prone.

The Accident-Prone Environment

A child's environment is usually more accident-prone than she is. Children will be children, and it is up to you, the parent, to shape your child's environment to reduce the possibility of accidents. Accidents often occur during the time a child is moving from one level of development to another, when parents' protective measures have not caught up with the child's new abilities. This chapter has suggestions for making your child's environment safer.

Childhood accidents often occur when there is a change from the usual familiar family routine. Watch for the following high-risk situations:

Family vacations

Moving into a new home

A change in caregivers or babysitters

High levels of stress in the family, such as during divorce or marital problems

A prolonged illness in one or both parents.

Accidents often occur when parents are tired or rushed and therefore less cautious. We have found it helpful when we start any new family adventure to take a few moments to think about what accidents may occur and warn ourselves to increase our vigilance at this time.

Develop a balance between protecting your child from accidents and educating her about safety. We used to take frequent trips to a summer cottage that was surrounded by rocks. We found it safer to take some time and climb the rocks with our preschoolers, showing them how to climb safely and what hazards to avoid. We designated where they were allowed to climb and where they were not to climb. When guests came, they simply told their children they were not to climb the rocks at all. As a result the children never developed the skills to climb safely, but they would try to sneak away from the watchful eyes of their parents and climb without supervision. Inevitably, accidents would happen. Don't be over-protective or under-protective; be wisely protective and help your child learn to protect herself.

How to Child-Proof Your Home

At each age and stage of your child's development anticipate possible accidents and shape your child's environment accordingly. Crawl around your house on your hands and knees, if you have to, and look for potential accident sources from your child's viewpoint. Have your older children help you and make it a family project. This teaches older children that they must learn to watch out for their younger siblings. Here are some things to watch for.

Toy safety.   Are small mouthable toy parts (e.g., Legos, Barbie doll shoes) lying on the floor? Teach older children not to leave these items within reach of baby.

Do you frequently check the safety of your child's toys? Look for broken or loose parts and sharp edges.

Medicines and other hazardous substances.   Do you have safety caps on all drugs or chemicals? Are they stored out of the reach of children, in locked cabinets? Do you *always* put the covers back on tightly? Don't leave an open bottle sitting within reach of a child while you are using it. Do you dispose of old medicines? Have you stored kerosine or gasoline cans in the garage or basement out of reach of the curious child?

You should have a poison prevention kit containing syrup of ipecac and activated charcoal in an accessible place. (See page 212.) Is the number of the nearest poison control center posted with other emergency numbers near your phone?

Around the house.   Do you keep plastic wrap, plastic bags, and balloons out of the reach of your children? Are hot radiator pipes covered? Are scissors, sewing tools, cigarette lighters, and guns out of reach? Are dangling cords, strings, and clothesline out of reach? Secure the dangling cords from window blinds or draperies a few feet up and out of reach.

Does your child chew on furniture? If the furniture is old (made before 1970), it may be covered with harmful lead-containing paint. Get rid of it. If your child is just beginning to walk, have you covered sharp edges (coffee table corners, fireplace bricks) with rubber protectors? We have found that adhesive-backed weather-stripping is useful for this. It is inexpensive, easy to apply, and easy to remove—though admittedly not very attractive.

Is there a small night light in your child's bedroom? Night lights prevent the drowsy child from banging into furniture and stumbling over toys during her nighttime trips to the bathroom.

Are electrical cords in good condition and out of reach so your baby cannot trip on them, chew on them, or use them to pull an appliance down on herself? Are unused electrical outlets covered with dummy plugs? Are electrical devices kept away from running water in the kitchen and bathroom?

Are windows properly locked? Are the screens secure? (Young children often like to lean against screens). If you have a screened window which is easily accessible, use screen guards to catch the screen in case your child pushes it open. Is there furniture in front of open windows? Children may climb on the furniture to get to the window. Do you have large visible decals on large panes of clear glass such as sliding doors? Children often don't see the glass and crash into or through it.

Are your stairs well lighted, not slippery, with safe handrails? Are the edges protected with rubber stripping or carpet? Teach your toddler how to back down stairs safely. Tack down loose carpeting and remove objects that children can trip over.

Do you have effective safety gates in front of stairs? Are your gates themselves safe? Children can get caught and strangle in the v-shaped tops of folding gates. Look for pressure gates with mesh that will not trap little fingers. When children start to climb over gates, they should no longer be used.

Fire safety. Is your home protected against fire? Are there smoke alarms appropriately placed about your house? Do you have working fire extinguishers in the most hazardous areas—the kitchen and the garage? Do you smoke in bed? Is the fireplace screen in place whenever the fireplace is in use?

Have you rehearsed a plan for escape in case of a fire? Does your child know how to get out by herself if she can't reach you? Designate a meeting place outside the house in case of a fire so you will know quickly if anyone is still inside.

Is your baby's nightwear flame-retardant? Stickers called "tot finders" are available from your local fire department. They should be placed on your children's bedroom doors and windows.

Bathroom safety.   Is your bathtub safe? Place non-skid bath mats or adhesive strips on the bottom of tubs and showers. Place a padded cover on the faucet. Make sure all bathroom rugs and mats have slip-proof backings.

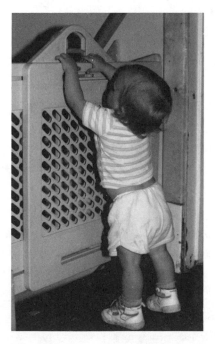

A safety gate at the top of the stairs will prevent falls.

Never leave young children alone in the bathtub. Do not fill the bathtub until you are ready to use it and drain it as soon as you've finished. Keep the door to the bathroom closed so your toddler won't wander in.

Is your hot water too hot? To avoid burns the hot water heater should be set no higher than 130°F (54°C).

In the kitchen. Are all glasses used by your child unbreakable? Do you turn pot handles toward the back of the stove? Are knives and appliances out of reach? Do you avoid giving foods that are easy to choke on to the child under three—nuts, orange seeds, raw carrot? Supervise your child closely if she is eating any of these foods. Children are more likely to choke if they are running around or are distracted while eating.

Outdoor safety. Is your yard safe? Have you removed boards with splinters and nails, toxic plants and berries, garden tools? Is the playground equipment sturdy and free of splinters and sharp corners? Are there rules for its safe use? Teach children not to walk in front of or behind a swing which is in use.

Swing sets and climbing equipment should be installed at least six feet away from obstructions such as fences or walls. The surface under them should be soft to absorb the force of falls; four to six inches' depth of pea gravel is a good shock absorber. Swing sets should be anchored firmly in the ground, and any exposed bolts or screws should be covered with plastic caps or taped over. Swings with chair, sling, or saddle seats are the safest because they discourage children from standing up and help them to hold their bodies on the swing. Place swings at different heights for children of different sizes.

Don't leave garden hoses lying in the sunshine. The water in the hose may become hot enough to scald the curious child. Do not use a power lawn mower while a child is in the yard.

Do you know, and have you pointed out to your child, which plants around your yard are potentially poisonous?

Has your child been instructed about not leaving the yard without permission?

If your child is a tree climber, have you surveyed the limbs to determine if any are weak or rotten? Have you told your child exactly which trees and limbs are off limits?

If you have a pool, is it properly fenced in? (See pages 196-198 for more on pool safety.) Do you empty your child's wading pool after use?

If you have an automatic garage door opener, caution your child against playing near the garage door when it is opening or closing. Outlaw games where children race under the closing door. Children have been pinned and crushed under closing garage doors. (They're not like elevator doors which open again if people get caught in them.) Keep automatic garage door openers out of the reach of children. Beginning at age two years, make frequent "do not touch" rounds through your house with your child, pointing out the hazards of dangerous substances and objects. Because toddlers have short memories and are impulsive, don't rely solely on this safety prevention education. There is no better way to keep your child safe than with adequate supervision.

Crib Safety

Crib accidents are one of the most common and serious injuries in infants and children. In 1974 the United States government enacted regulations governing cribs and cradles; these standards were revised in 1979. Be wary of cribs manufactured before 1974. Be sure that they conform to the safety standards listed below. Pamphlets concerning crib safety are available from the U.S. Consumer Product Safety Commission. Call the hotline at 1-800-638-8326; Maryland only, 1-800-492-8363; Alaska, Hawaii, Puerto Rico, and the Virgin Islands, 1-800-638-8333. In Canada ask for the pamphlet "Are You Sure Your Crib Is Safe?" from Consumer and Corporate Affairs, Department of Product Safety, 1410 Stanley Street, Montreal, Quebec H3A 1P8; phone 1-514-283-2825.

Safety Standards for Cribs

Cribs should be painted with lead-free paint. Those manufactured after 1974 should conform to the government regulations that specify lead-free paint. Those manufactured prior to 1974 may have been repainted several times with lead-containing paint; if this is the case, don't use the crib. If your child is a chewer, cover the guard rails with non-toxic ''chew-guards.''

Mattresses. The mattress should fit the crib perfectly. An undersized mattress will leave a gap along the side or end of the crib where an infant's head can get caught, causing suffocation. To check the fit of a crib mattress, push it into one corner. There should be no more than a one-and-a-half-inch (3.8 cm) gap between it and the side or end of the crib. If you can fit more than two fingers between the mattress and the crib, the mattress is too small. Beware of hand-me-down or second-hand cribs in which the mattress may be different from the one designed to fit this crib exactly.

Make sure the four metal hangers supporting the mattress and support board are secured into their notches by safety clips or safety plugs. Check the support system regularly by rattling the metal hangers and by pushing the mattress from the top and then from the bottom. If a hanger support dislodges, it needs to be fixed or replaced. Avoid floating mattress support designs. These hooks can become detached, causing the mattress to collapse at one corner. Babies can slide into the gap between the mattress and frame and strangle. Fixed mattress supports or non-slip hooks are much safer.

Avoid loose plastic mattress covers or waterproof sheets. They can wrap around a baby's head and cause suffocation. Never leave a baby unattended on a water bed. Infants have suffocated on water beds.

Height of sides. When the height of the side rail is less than three-quarters of a baby's height, she can no longer be safely left alone in the crib. If the baby can get her chin above the crib rail with the mattress placed in the lowest position, she is too tall to be left alone in the crib. A child who is 35 inches in height has outgrown the crib and should sleep in a bed. As a general guide the distance between the mattress in its lowest position and the top of the side rails should be at least 26 inches (66 cm). When the mattress is in its highest position, the top of the lowered crib rail should remain at least nine inches (22.8 cm) above the mattress support.

Are the drop sides secure? To prevent babies from accidently releasing the drop sides, each one should be secured with two locking devices. Some cribs have a spring-type locking device on either side of the rail and a foot bar release at the bottom of the rail. If your crib only has one locking device, you can install another by adding a slide bolt at one end of the drop side. The infant should not be able to release the drop sides from inside the crib.

Spacing of bars. The maximum distance between the bars of the crib rail should be 2-3/8 inches (6 cm), so that babies cannot get their heads caught between the bars. The bars of cribs made prior to 1979 may have wider spacing that does not conform to these standards.

Where to put the crib. The crib should not be placed against a window, near any dangling cords from blinds or draperies, or near any furniture which could be used to help the infant climb out. Give some thought to what could happen if your baby does climb out of the crib: the crib should be placed so that she will not fall against any sharp object or become entrapped and possibly strangle between the crib and an adjacent wall or piece of furniture.

Bumpers and toys. Bumpers should run around the entire crib, tie or snap into place, and have at least six straps. To prevent your baby from chewing on the straps or becoming entangled in them, trim off any excess length. Remove bumpers and toys from the crib as soon as a child begins to pull herself up on the crib rails. Bumpers and toys can be used as steps for climbing over the rail. Toys, mobiles, pacifiers, and clothing worn in the crib should not have strings longer than than eight inches. Strings can strangle. Remove mobiles and crib exercisers when baby begins to sit up.

Other safety points.   Avoid cribs with decorative cut-outs and knobs. A baby's clothes or the ties and strings on them can get caught on these projections, causing strangulation. Knobs and posts can be sawed off and the tops sanded smooth. Avoid cribs with ornate tops. Infants have strangled in the concave space between the posts and the crib. Never tie or harness a child in a crib. Be sure there are no elastics, scarves, necklaces, or loose cords anywhere in the crib that could wrap around the baby's neck. Buttons on clothing can become entangled in the mesh of a mesh crib or playpen.

Check the crib hardware for sharp points or edges and holes or cracks where your baby's fingers could get pinched or stuck.

If the baby's room is not within hearing distance of every room of the house (mothers have exceptionally good hearing), an intercom may prove to be a valuable safety feature. A baby should not be left unattended with a propped-up bottle.

If you are giving or selling your crib to someone else, make sure it's in safe condition and that the original instructions are passed on to the new owner. It is illegal to sell a crib that does not meet government regulations. In some countries, it is illegal to sell a crib without its instructions.

Safety while sharing sleep.   During the baby and toddler years, many parents find that the whole family sleeps best if the baby or young child sleeps with the parents. This is especially true if the mother is breastfeeding. It is safe for parents to sleep with their baby or child. Pushing the bed against the wall or using a guard rail will protect the baby from falls. The baby is probably safer between the mother and the guard rail than between the mother and the father, since the mother, even while sleeping, is more aware of the baby's presence and needs. Parents who are under the influence of sedative medication, drugs, or alcohol—anything which decreases awareness—should not take their babies to bed with them.

How to Buy Safe Baby Equipment

Baby Carriers
I strongly advise parents to "wear" their baby. This enhances bonding between infant and parents, reduces crying, and increases your overall enjoyment of your baby. The custom of wearing your baby fits in beautifully with today's busy lifestyles. You'll find that a baby carrier will take you places you can't go with a stroller: up and down steps, over hiking trails, between the racks of a crowded department store. And you'll get there with less aggravation.

Safety. Choose only a carrier made by a reputable manufacturer. There are a great many baby carriers being introduced, and I fear that some of them have not been adequately safety-tested. Be sure the straps and connectors are sturdy and properly attached. The leg openings should be large enough not to pinch but small enough to keep the infant from falling out. The carrier should be deep enough to support the head of a baby under six months, and deep enough to support her back when older than six months. Periodically check for frayed straps, loose hardware, or ripped seams.

Comfort. Baby carriers should be comfortable for both parents and baby. Cotton or a cotton-polyester blend is the most comfortable fabric. It also washes well. A well-designed baby carrier should distribute the baby's weight on the shoulders and hips of the adult, not on the back and neck. You should be able to stand normally while using it without arching your back or leaning forward. It should be well padded at the shoulders. Padding along the edges that press against baby's torso and legs makes the carrier more comfortable for baby. To avoid having to purchase a series of carriers, choose one that can be adjusted to various carrying positions as your baby gets older.

Ease of use.   Human nature dictates that if something is not convenient to use, it won't get used very often. Fathers especially shy away from carriers that have many sets of buckles and straps that have to be adjusted with each use. A carrier that can be adjusted or removed while the baby is in it prevents unnecessary disturbances. Mothers should be able to breastfeed discreetly without

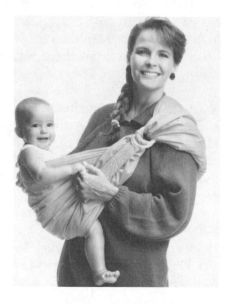

A sling-type carrier is versatile and convenient to use.

removing the baby from the carrier. Look for a carrier that is nice-looking, in a color that complements your wardrobe so that you will feel good about using it.

Types of carriers.   In my experience a sling-type carrier is usually the most versatile for accommodating a baby's changing size and development. In the early months, the infant can be cradled securely against mother's chest, making breastfeeding easy. Later on, the child can be carried on the hip. The sling distributes the baby's weight between the parent's shoulder and hip, placing less strain on the back. Baby carriers serve many purposes; they provide nurturing, convenience, and fun.

Infant Seats

Falls out of infant seats are one of the most common accidents in the early months of life. Do not leave a baby unattended in a seat that is placed on a table or a counter top, not even "just for a second" while you do something else. By three months of age, a baby is able to roll out of an infant seat. When babies are around five or six months, they may rock forward in the seat and topple over sideways. It is safest to place the infant seat on a cushioned surface, preferably the floor. Other safety tips:

Use the restraining belts.

Be sure that the infant seat has a wide, sturdy base with supporting devices that fasten securely to keep the seat from collapsing.

Be sure that the supporting bars are fastened securely. If they pop out of the sockets the seat will fall backwards.

Attach non-skid tape to the supports to prevent slipping.

Do not use an infant seat as a substitute for a car seat.

High Chairs

High chairs should have a wide base for stability. Be sure the chair and tray are free of sharp edges and splinters. Keep the chair away from hazards such as stoves and ovens. Use the safety belt, and be sure the belt is attached to the frame and not the tray. Do not depend on the tray to restrain the child. Be sure the tray is properly latched on both sides. Children tend to push against the tray when seated or pull on the tray when climbing into the chair.

Toddlers and preschoolers like to climb up on high chairs from the floor. This should be done only with supervision, as most high chairs will topple over if they are not secured by an adult.

Playpens

The safety tips that apply to cribs apply to playpens as well. The distance between the slats should be the same as a crib. If using a mesh playpen, the netting should be small enough that it cannot catch the buttons on a child's clothing. Avoid mesh with large openings, which make easy toe holes for climbing. *Never* leave a child in a mesh playpen with the side down. A child can become trapped and can strangle in the pocket of mesh between the floor of the playpen and the lowered side.

Avoid putting anything on or in the playpen that has strings longer than eight inches. Remove large toys or boxes that can be used as steps for climbing out. Cover exposed nuts and bolts. Secure latching mechanisms that may act like scissors and pinch baby's fingers.

Strollers

Look for strollers that are safe, stable, and sturdy. Strollers really take a beating, so look for one that will stand up to wear and tear.

The stroller base should be wide, with the rear wheels well behind the weight of the child so that it will not tip when baby leans over the side or rocks backwards. If the stroller adjusts to a reclining position, be sure that it will not tip backward when the baby is lying down. Shopping baskets should be placed directly over or in front of the rear axle to prevent tipping.

Brakes on two wheels are safer than single brakes. Be sure that latching devices fasten securely. Latches can be accidentally tripped, causing the stroller to collapse, so strollers with two latching devices holding them open are safer than those with only one. Be careful of fingers— yours and the baby's—when collapsing or opening a stroller. Check the stroller for sharp edges.

Walkers

Though many infants enjoy walkers, I do not encourage their use because of the safety hazards and the possibility of confusing an infant's development of locomotive skills. Infants develop from the head down. Development of motor skills in the upper half of their body always precedes the development of those in the lower half. Walkers reverse this process: they provide the lower half of the body with a means of locomotion that the mind and upper half are not yet ready for. A few minutes a day of supervised play in a walker will not harm your baby, but it should not be used without supervision.

Since walkers tip easily, be sure the wheel base is much larger than the frame that holds the baby. A properly designed walker should not tip when baby leans over the side to look at something on the floor. Be sure the wheels are sturdy. Flimsy wheels may bend, causing tipping.

Be sure all coiled springs and hinges are encased in protective covers. Avoid the older x-frame walkers which can pinch fingers.

Remove throw rugs and other obstacles which may become entangled in the wheels and cause the walker to tip. Do not rely on gates to prevent falls down the stairs. An impetuous infant may get up enough momentum to crash right through the gate. Do not let your child go exploring on her own in the walker as she is able to get into potential hazards she would otherwise be unable to reach.

Choosing Safe Toys

The safety of a toy depends on its design, how it is made, and the age and skills of the children using it. Recommended ages on toy packages provide only the most general guidelines for toy safety. Use your discretion and your knowledge of your child when selecting toys. Be careful when a younger child plays with toys meant for an older sibling. Toys should fit your child's developmental stage and temperament. If your child is a thrower, get her soft, lightweight toys. Missile-type toys (darts and arrows) can cause eye injuries. If your child is a tearer and biter, avoid foam-rubber toys which can be easily bitten or torn apart and swallowed.

Children under three who still put things in their mouths should not be given toys with small, removable parts which could be swallowed. Check that eyes and other features on stuffed animals are securely fastened. The tiny noisemakers in squeeze-and-squeak toys should be non-removable. Avoid squeak toys with flared handles which can lodge in a child's throat and cause suffocation. Rattles should have a head no less than 1-3/8 inches by 2 inches (3.5 cm by 5 cm). Toys for babies should be at least 1-3/8 inches in diameter to avoid swallowing and choking.

Be careful of crib toys—toys which are fastened between the two side rails and hang over the crib, giving infants something to look at and reach for. These toys are recommended only from birth to five months, and should definitely be removed when the infant is old enough to push up on hands and knees. Toys with strings longer than eight inches are dangerous.

Cloth toys should be labeled flame-retardant or non-flammable. Avoid poorly constructed dolls and animals stuffed with small loose pellets that will fall out when the seams tear open. Avoid thin plastic toys which are likely to break easily, leaving sharp or jagged edges. Flex the plastic slightly to see if it is brittle. Be sure that painted toys are labeled ''non-toxic.''

Be careful of balloons. It is wise not to give balloons to a child under three. Caution children not to put balloons in their mouths. Uninflated balloons may cause choking. The pieces left when a balloon pops are also hazardous. Gather them up and throw them out immediately to keep babies and young children from putting the pieces in their mouths. Dispose of large plastic bags and other plastic wrappers when unpacking toys, as this material can also cause suffocation.

Toy Storage
Avoid toy chests with attached lids that can fall on the child, causing injury and strangulation. Hinged lids should stay open by themselves, without propping. Toy shelves are much safer and teach the developing infant and child a sense of order. Visit a local Montessori School and you will notice the wise use of toy shelves with separate compartments for individual toys.

Toy Safety and the Law
According to Public Law 91-113, the Bureau of Product Safety can require that unsafe toys be removed from retailers' shelves. This law also gives you the right to return any toys on the Bureau's hazardous toy list for full reimbursement. If you purchase any items that you find hazardous, write: Consumer Product Safety Commission, Washington DC, 20207. Describe the article completely, where it was purchased, its country of origin, and what part of the toy is hazardous. Include your name, address, and phone number. If you require a current list of hazardous toys, baby furniture, and other baby products, call the Consumer Product Safety Commission's toll-free hotline at 1-800-638-8326; Maryland only, 1-800-492-8363; Alaska, Hawaii, Puerto Rico, and the Virgin Islands, 1-800-638-8333. In Canada contact: Consumer and Corporate Affairs, Department of Product Safety, 1410 Stanley Street, Montreal, Quebec H3A 1P8; phone 1-514-283-2825.

Car Safety

I cannot overemphasize the importance of safely secur-
ing your infant or child in an approved car seat while driving. I have seen the tragic results of removing an infant
from a car seat in order to comfort her or of not placing
the child in the car seat "because we are only traveling
a few blocks." Fortunately most states now have laws re-
quiring the use of safety seats and seat belts. Observe the
following car safety tips:

Never let your baby ride in your arms while the car is
moving.

Always use a government-approved crash-tested car
seat for infants and young children. Always follow
the manufacturer's directions for use.

Attach the car safety belt to the car seat correctly.
Make sure it is firm and tight.

Use a top tether strap if one is required.

Use the safety belt, harness, and/or shield in the car
seat as directed.

Do not strap two children or a parent and a child into
one seat belt.

Do not allow children to play with sharp objects such
as pencils or metal toys while the car is moving.
These objects become dangerous projectiles if the
car stops suddenly.

Choose a car seat appropriate for your child's age and
weight.

Do not use an infant carrier or infant seat in a car as a
substitute for a car seat.

Do not use a travel bed in a car.

Do not wear your baby in a cloth carrier in the car.

Always insist that older children use seat belts.

Always wear a seat belt yourself.

Choosing and Using the Right Car Seat

There are a variety of car seats on the market in a range of prices. Some are appropriate for infants, some for older children, and some can be adjusted as the child grows.

Infants from birth to twenty pounds. Car seats for infants of this age and weight are designed so that the infant faces the back of the car and reclines at a 45° angle. The car seat is secured so that most of the forward force of a collision is transmitted to the seat belt holding the seat. The rear-facing, semi-upright position allows the remaining force to be distributed throughout the baby's back, to bones and muscles. A safety harness secures the baby in the seat.

There are two general types of car seats for infants of this age and weight: tub-like and convertible. The tub-like seats are only for infants weighing less than 20 pounds. They are simple, lightweight, less expensive, and can be used to transport a sleeping baby outside the car. The convertible type of car seat can be turned forward when baby weighs more than twenty pounds and can be used for the next couple of years, until the child is big enough for a lap belt. Convertible car seats are heavier and more expensive, but they can be used longer; you do not have to buy a second car seat when your child is older.

Your baby is ready to graduate from the backward-facing to the forward-facing position when she can sit alone without support, weighs at least 18 to 20 pounds, and is restless in the backward position.

Car seats for infants weighing 20 to 40 pounds. Seats for older babies and young children come in two basic types: the traditional car seat, either a convertible as mentioned above, or a seat purchased especially for this size child; or the seat with a booster cushion and a protective shield secured by the car's lap belt, for older toddlers and preschoolers.

The booster seat is one of the easiest car-safety devices to use, if your child is disciplined enough to stay in it. The main disadvantage of this type of car seat is that it has poor side protection, and children can slip out of it very easily. Check the manufacturer's directions for how big a child must be to use this seat safely.

The more traditional car seat, either the convertible type that was used for the tiny infant or one that was purchased especially for this age and weight group, is safer for most children. The side protection is better, and the safety harness keeps the child in the seat. These seats are a little less easy to use than the protective shield. They are not as easy to secure in the car, and some models require a top tether strap to prevent them from pitching forward.

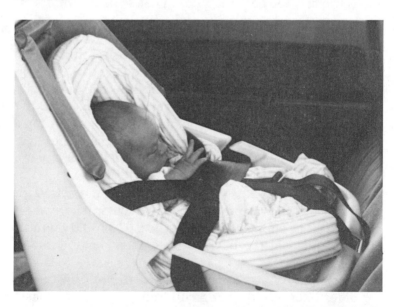

A folded sling baby carrier helps to support and cushion the tiny infant in a car seat.

Older children. Children over 40 pounds (and usually over four years of age) can ride on a firm cushion just high enough to allow the car's lap belt to ride across their hips with the lower edge of the belt touching their thighs. The seat belt should be at an angle of 45° for maximum safety. The seat belt should not ride above the hip bones because the force of impact in a collision would then be transferred to the abdominal organs rather than to the hip bones. Shoulder belts may not fit the small, restless child properly. If the shoulder belt crosses the child's body above the chest, at her neck, she is too small to use it. A properly fitting shoulder belt should cross the child's shoulder at the collarbone. If the shoulder belt does not fit the child properly, put it behind her back and use the lap belt only. Lap belts alone are not recommended for children under the age of four or those who weigh less than 40 pounds. These children should be in a safety seat.

Tips for Safe and Pleasant Car Travel
Theoretically, the center of the rear seat is the safest place for a child in a car safety seat. Practically speaking, parents traveling alone with a child frequently take their eyes off the road and turn around to check that the child in the back seat is all right. An easily distracted parent may be better off putting the child in the front passenger seat. Although it is not as safe a place, it may be more conducive to safe driving.

Be careful not to place your child's bare skin against the hot plastic of the car seat if your car has been sitting in the hot sun. This is a common cause of burns during hot weather. Car seat covers protect the baby's skin against hot or cold surfaces and cushion the baby as well. Rolled blankets, towels, or diapers on each side of baby help to support wobbly heads and increase comfort. A folded baby sling makes an ideal horseshoe-shaped head support for a tiny infant in the car seat. To prevent chafing, be sure your baby is clothed in areas where the harness strap passes over her body.

Do not try to place your baby in a car seat with a blanket wrapped around her. The harness will not fit correctly over the shoulders. If the baby needs the extra warmth, cut holes in the blanket for the harness and crotch strap. Put the blanket in the seat, pull the straps through the holes, place the baby in the seat, buckle the harness, and then fold the blanket over the baby.

Don't leave the rear door of a hatch-back or station wagon open when you have passengers in the back seat. This lets in exhaust fumes, and dangerous objects may come through the open door in the event of a crash. Children should never ride in the luggage compartment of hatch-backs or in the cargo areas of pick-up trucks or vans. Secure car doors and tail gates with safety latches, if available.

Keeping order in the car pool. Insist upon strict obedience to rules when you have several children in the car. Encourage desirable behavior right from the start, before undesirable behavior turns the car into a moving wrestling ring. Songs, word games, riddles, and interesting stories will usually hold young children's attention for a short period of time. When the car comes to a stop and you are dropping off a child, insist that an adult get out first to ensure that there are no oncoming vehicles. Only then should the child be allowed to open her door and get out. To avoid catching fingers in slamming car doors, insist that the doors be closed by an adult. Agree to carry no more passengers than you have seat belts. In an emergency, three children can be protected with two seat belts in the back seat by having the child in the middle share the belts of the children on either side. In other words, the left-side seat belt is fastened around the child on the left and the child in the middle, and the right-side seat belt is fastened around the child on the right and the child in the middle. Research shows that three children sharing two belts in this way are safer than two children in one belt.

All pregnant mothers should use seat belts. Until your child is born, you are his or her "car seat." Your behavior is protecting two lives. Keep the lap belt below your uterus, across the pelvic bone, to avoid injury to your baby from the seat belt in the event of a crash. You and your baby are safer in a seat belt than you would be if thrown from the car or into the dashboard in a collision.

Make your baby's first ride a safe ride. If baby rides home from the hospital in an approved car seat and never travels in a car without one, it becomes part of the habit of car travel. There should be no exceptions to the rule about putting your infant and child in the proper car seat. Some infants and children may strongly protest being restrained in the car seat. Our family has been through 22 years of car travel with six children of varied temperaments. We have discovered some solutions to the crying-baby-in-the-car-seat dilemma. If your tiny infant hates the car seat, as often as possible, travel with two adults in the car. One adult sits in the back next to the baby in the car seat (and uses a seat belt) while the other adult drives. Even in the car the breast is a source of comfort. It's possible for a nursing mother to position herself to breastfeed her baby in a rear-facing car seat while remaining buckled-in herself. Above all resist the temptation to take a crying baby out of the car seat for comforting. Wait until you can stop the car. Safety comes before psychology in this situation. There's nothing wrong with stopping the car for a few minutes to comfort a crying baby. It may take longer to get where you're going, but almost everything takes longer once you have children. An older sibling can help to distract and entertain a baby who is unhappy about being in a car seat. Songs work well, and you can make them up to fit the situation:

I don't like my car seat,
I don't like my car seat,
It makes me be as quiet as a mousie.

Water Safety

We have always enjoyed water sports as our main mode of family recreation. We have taught our children to respect water—both its pleasures and its dangers. The U. S. Consumer Product Safety Commission estimates that each year 260 children under five years of age drown in residential swimming pools and spas. Another three thousand children under five are treated in hospital emergency rooms following submersion accidents each year. Some of these accidents result in permanent brain damage. In warm-weather states, drowning is the leading cause of accidental death in children under five.

Pool and spa areas should be enclosed with a fence and a self-latching, self-closing gate. The latch should be on the inside of the gate well beyond the child's reach. Although most states have laws about enclosing pools with fences, some families enclose the entire backyard. Neighboring children may be protected from your pool, but your own child may not be. Spas are particularly dangerous since warm-water drowning becomes serious more quickly. Unfenced spas should be covered with a rigid safety cover.

Keep the pool covered in the months it isn't in use. The newer rigid covers are safer than the flexible covers or solar blankets. Never use a pool with its cover partially in place, since children may become trapped under it. Remove the cover completely when your pool is in use.

Never leave a child unsupervised near a pool. Instruct babysitters about potential hazards to young children in and around swimming pools and the need for constant supervision. You may wish to limit your child's swimming to times when parents, rather than babysitters, can supervise. Flotation devices are no substitute for supervision. Teach your child never to play in a pool away from home without your approval and adult supervision. One-third of all childhood drownings occur in the pools of neighbors.

Place tables and chairs well away from the pool fence to prevent children from climbing into the pool area. Keep toys away from the pool area, because a young child playing with the toys could accidently topple into the water. Remove steps to above-ground pools when not in use.

Install a telephone at poolside to avoid the temptation to leave children unattended in or near the pool to answer the phone inside the house. Keep emergency numbers at the poolside telephone. The most recent near-drowning case in my practice occurred when a mother left the pool area to answer the telephone. The three-year-old rode his tricycle into the pool, nearly drowned, was resuscitated by paramedics, but now has permanent severe brain damage. It is better to let the phone ring than leave a child unattended near a pool.

Keep rescue equipment near the pool. This should include a floatable pole longer than one-half the pool's width, a ring buoy attached to a rope, and a first-aid kit. Next to this kit post a list of emergency phone numbers and a poster showing cardiopulmonary resuscitation. These are usually available at pool supply stores. Pool owners should have updated knowledge of CPR.

If you have lighting installed in and around the pool, be sure this lighting is UL-approved and installed by a competent electrician.

Diving accidents can result in paralysis from injury to the neck when the head hits the side or bottom of the pool. Teach your child to observe the following precautions:

Never dive into above-ground pools.

Don't dive in the shallow end of an in-ground pool. Enter the water feet first. Dive only from the end of the diving board or the deep end of the pool.

Dive with your hands in front of you and immediately steer your body upward to avoid hitting the bottom or sides of the pool.

In using a pool slide, never slide down head first.

If you have a backyard pool or your family enjoys water sports, it is wise to teach your infant to swim. Even one-year-old babies can learn to keep their heads above water for ten seconds, although this does not mean that they are safe from drowning. An excellent source is the book *How to Teach Your Baby to Swim*, by Claire Timmermans (New York: Stein and Day, 1984). Swimming lessons are not a substitute for parental supervision.

Boating Safety

Boats require additional discipline. If you are a boating family, teach your child at a very young age that boating means wearing a life jacket. There are no exceptions. If you begin when your child is young and if you are firm, your child will accept the rule. Unfortunately, many of the life jackets approved by the Coast Guard are cumbersome, and many children refuse to wear them. Attempt to fit your child with a floatation device that she will accept, and introduce this as a requirement for boating. The life jacket should be one that automatically keeps your child's head above water. Besides a personal floatation device, a leash and safety harness may be used to protect a roving toddler on a boat.

We have taken frequent sailing trips with our children over the years. Before embarking my wife and I set down strict boating rules. The older children are to keep watch on the younger ones, and everyone wears a life jacket at all times. We rehearse a man-overboard drill, and there is no horse play. We have taught our children both to enjoy and respect the sea.

Cycle Safety

I remember when the term ''motor milestone'' referred to the time when a child crawled, walked, or ran. In today's mobile world, motor milestones may refer to a child's progression from walker, to tricycle, to bicycle (with anywhere from one to eighteen speeds), and then— heaven forbid!—to Moped or motorcycle. All this cycling requires a keen eye for safety.

Choosing and Maintaining a Safe Bike

Be sure the bike fits the child. When your child is sitting on the seat with hands on the handlebars, he or she must be able to place the balls of both feet on the ground. Boys should be able to straddle the center bar with both feet flat on the ground and one inch of clearance between the crotch and the bar. Adjust handlebar grips so that they are at a comfortable height and at right angles to the handlebar stem. Children tend to overestimate the size bike they need, perhaps expressing their own need to be bigger. Start small and work up. Remind your child that she will have a bigger bike when she is bigger. Here's a checklist for choosing a safe bicycle:

Does the bike meet the required federal safety standards?

Exposed bolts should have protective covers.

The bike should have side, rear, and front reflectors.

Handlebars should have hand grips. The cross bar in the center of the handlebars should be padded.

Coaster brakes are usually safer than hand brakes for the young child.

Avoid bikes with high-rise handlebars and small wheels. These are difficult for the young child to control.

Pedals should have rough surfaces and guards which prevent the feet from slipping off.

Periodically check your child's bike for loose wheels, bolts, chain guards, seats, and especially handlebars. Test the brakes and check that the tires are properly inflated.

Cycling Rules of the Road

Impress upon your child that bicycles driven in traffic are subject to the same laws and traffic control signals as mo-

tor vehicles. Children should come to a full stop at inter-
sections and walk the bike across rather than ride. Ride
with the traffic, not against it, always keeping on the right-
hand edge of the road. Ride in single file. Use arm signals to indicate stops and turns. When riding past parked
cars, be on the alert for car doors opening and for cars
pulling out into traffic.

Discourage riding at night, but if it is necessary, insist
that your child wear ankle lights which produce a moving warning light. Reflectors should be visible from all
sides. Reflectorized orange vests, like those used by hunt-
ers, provide additional protection for night cyclers.

Test brakes frequently. If the bike has hand brakes, be
sure it has both front and rear brakes. Encourage your
child to apply brakes gently, favoring the rear brake first.
Use extra caution when braking and riding on slippery
surfaces. Don't ride fast downhill.

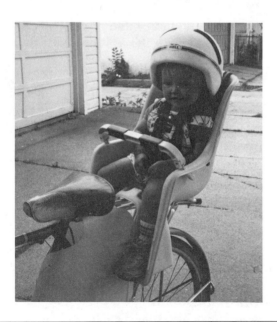

Children riding in carriers on adult bicycles
should wear safety helmets.

Cycling with Infants and Small Children
Do not carry infants under six months on a bicycle. They
are unable to sit up, and their heads may be too wobbly.
Use a backpack for infants six to twelve months. Children from one to four should be carried in a special child-
carrier seat which is mounted over the rear wheel of an
adult bicycle. It has built-in safety harnesses and foot rests
which keep the child's feet away from the spokes. Always
put a safety helmet on your young passenger. Ride only
on bike paths or safe streets, not in busy traffic.

Protecting Your Child from Dangerous Strangers

Parents today worry about kidnapping, child molestation,
and sexual abuse. You can't be with your child every mo-
ment, so you must teach her, at an early age, what to do
to keep herself safe.

Build up a trusting relationship with your child so that
she feels comfortable telling you secrets. She should feel
that she can tell you anything. Beginning at age three, remind her that she can tell mommy or daddy about something she has done or something she is worried about, and
you will not get angry. Use words and actions that she
will understand and that will make her feel comfortable
when she tells you something. Child molesters often tell
their victims not to tell their parents and threaten them
with the loss of parental love if they do; your child should
know that this will not happen.

Teach your child the meaning of "private parts" and
that no one has the right to touch her in her private parts.
Tell her that there are good touches and bad touches. Good
touches make you feel good, bad touches make you feel
frightened. Your child has the right to tell someone that
she does not want to be touched. Tell her that if anyone
touches her in a way that makes her feel frightened, she
should tell mommy or daddy.

Teach your child about secrets. Tell her that she should
tell you if anyone asks her to keep a secret. Teach her the

difference between bad secrets and good secrets. If anyone gives her bad touches and asks her not to tell mommy
and daddy, those are bad secrets, and she should tell you
about those. Good secrets are things like what someone
is getting as a birthday present. Those are secrets she can
keep. If anyone offers her candy or money or wants to
take her picture, she should tell you, especially if that person tells her not to tell her parents.

Teach your child what a stranger is: someone she does
not know well. Uncle Harry and Aunt Nancy are not
strangers, but anyone your child does not know well, even
if it's someone from church or a classmate's parent, is a
stranger. Tell her never to go home with a stranger and
never to get in a stranger's car, even if that stranger says
that he or she will take the child to mommy or daddy.
If someone other than a parent is picking a child up after
school, the teacher should know about it. A child should
walk home from school with other children.

If a stranger stops and asks for directions, don't get
into the car to show him or her how to get somewhere.
If a child is lost in a store, she should not seek help from
a stranger, but should go to a cash register and find a sales
person. Teach your child to run into a busy place where
there are lots of people or into a neighbor's house or a
store if she is being followed. Tell her not to hide in a
secluded place such as an alley or the woods. She should
yell for help if a stranger is following her or grabbing her.
If your child is home alone, she should not let anyone inside the house, for any reason. Be sure that your child
knows how to use the telephone at home, as well as a pay
phone, and knows how to dial 911 or to dial the operator
for help in an emergency.

Be aware of signs of sexual abuse, in your children and
in other children. These include sudden changes in behavior, fear of leaving you, fear of being washed during
a bath, or a sudden fear of going to visit a previously
trusted friend or relative. Be aware that in most cases of
sexual abuse, the abuser is someone the child already
knows.

CHAPTER 11

First-Aid Procedures for Common Emergencies and Injuries

An important part of parenting your child is knowing what to do in an emergency. This chapter contains information about the most common childhood emergencies and injuries, with the most serious at the beginning. Your quick action can make your child more comfortable, prevent serious consequences, and may even save his life.

CPR

It is advisable for all parents and caregivers to take a certified course in cardiopulmonary resuscitation (CPR), usually given by your local hospital or Red Cross. It is wise to take a refresher course every few years, too. Junior-high and high-school-age children should also take CPR, especially if they frequently babysit for younger children. The following are step-by-step directions for CPR in children.

What to Do When a Child Stops Breathing

Step 1. Shout for help. A neighbor or passerby who hears you should call the paramedics. If you are all alone, start mouth-to-mouth breathing first for a few minutes, and then stop long enough to dial 911 or the operator for help.

Step 2. Clear the mouth. Look for foreign objects, gum, or food. Carefully remove anything you find with your finger. If there is vomit or other fluid in the mouth, turn the child on one side and use gravity to clear it. If you suspect choking, apply back blows as described in the section on choking (see page 208).

Step 3. Straighten the airway. Place child on his back. Bend (flex) the neck forward and extend the head backward so that the nose is tilted upward in a "sniffing" position. The head of a teenager or adult could be extended quite far backward. The head of an infant or small child should be extended only slightly, as too much extension

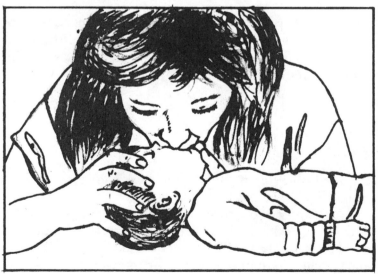

Mouth-to-mouth breathing for an infant

will obstruct the breathing. A towel rolled up under the neck usually maintains the correct position. If a neck injury is suspected, do not move the neck.

Step 4. Begin mouth-to-mouth breathing. Place one hand under the child's neck and the other on the forehead. In an infant under one year, cover the child's nose and mouth with your mouth. In older children squeeze the nostrils shut between your thumb and forefinger and fit your mouth tightly around the child's lips. Blow into the mouth with just enough force to see the chest rise when you blow. Begin with two short breaths. Give steady breaths, one every three seconds (20 breaths per minute) in an infant or toddler; one every four seconds (15 breaths per minute) in an older child; one every five seconds (12 breaths per minute) in teens and adults. Blow only enough air to make the chest move up and down.

If the chest does not move when you blow air into the mouth, check again for an obstruction in the airway. Continue mouth-to-mouth breathing until trained help arrives or until the child resumes breathing on his own.

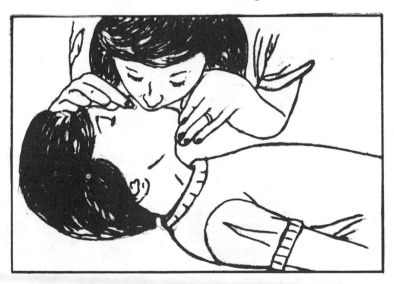

Mouth-to-mouth breathing for a child

What to Do When a Child's Heart Stops

Step 1. Check for a pulse. The easiest places to find a pulse in an infant are the groin (femoral pulse), the neck on either side of the Adam's apple (carotid artery), and the upper arm (brachial pulse). Checking the neck is the easiest way to find a pulse in an older child or adult. Usually you can see and feel the heartbeat of an infant and child by placing your hand over the left chest. If there is no pulse, go on to step 2.

Step 2. Start chest compressions. Place child on a firm surface—a table or the floor. In the infant, place two fingers on the middle one-third of the breast bone and depress the bone one-half to one inch at a rate of 100 times a minute. Compressing the heart of a newborn is easiest if you encircle the entire chest with your two hands and compress the breast bone with your two thumbs. In the older child depress the lower one-third of the breast bone with the heel of your hand at a rate of eighty compressions per minute. Give mouth-to-mouth puffs of air after every five compressions. Count it out for yourself

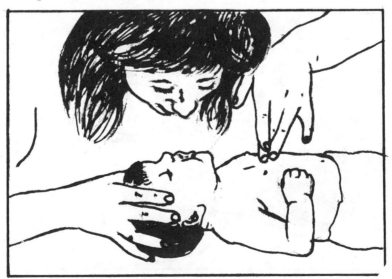

Chest compressions for an infant

as you do it: one, two, three, four, five—breath; one, two, three, four, five—breath.

Step 3. After five minutes, check pulse. Continue CPR, checking for a pulse every five minutes, until the child's heartbeat resumes, or until emergency help arrives.

Choking

Step 1. Be sure the child is really choking. If the child can speak, cry, cough, is not turning blue, and is obviously breathing, the airway is not obstructed, and you should not interfere with his own efforts to dislodge the material. The child's own cough reflex will usually handle the problem. Give him emotional support so he does not panic. The most common reason for efforts at clearing the throat is fluid that has gone down the wrong way.

If the child is trying to get a breath, but is making no sound, the airway is probably obstructed. Other signs of choking are a blue color, loss of consciousness, a wide-open mouth, excessive drooling, and panic. The older child

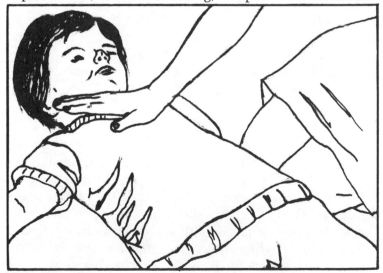

Chest compressions for a child

may grab the front of the throat with both hands; this is called the universal choking signal. Remember, if the child's airway is totally obstructed he is making no sound. It takes air to make noise. A foreign object in the airway may cause a partial obstruction, but still allow air to get through. If the child's efforts to clear a partial obstruction are not succeeding, seek medical help.

Step 2. Four back blows. If a child's airway is obstructed, hold him head down over your knee and forearm and administer four quick, hard blows on the back between the shoulder blades. Hold an infant face down on your forearm with the head and neck stabilized and your hand securely on the diaper area.

Step 3. Four chest thrusts. If the child's airway is still obstructed, flip the child over on his back and administer four chest thrusts. With the child lying on the floor or across your lap, place your hands across the front and sides of the child's lower chest. Quickly compress the abdomen upward with a thrust of the arms and hands. Repeat this three more times. The back blow procedure gives a higher instantaneous expelling pressure than the chest thrust, but chest thrusts are more sustained. The combination of back blows and chest thrusts will usually dislodge the foreign object. If this does not work, repeat both procedures again.

Step 4. Check for the object. If after back blows and chest thrusts, you can see the foreign object in the child's mouth and are certain you can get your finger around it, use your finger to remove it. Do not use a blind finger sweep to dislodge foreign bodies from the back of a child's throat. Inserting a large adult finger in a child's small throat can push the foreign body farther back into the throat or may cause the child to panic and suck the object into the lungs rather than swallow the object.

The Heimlich maneuver. Because of the danger of damage to abdominal organs the Heimlich maneuver is generally not recommended for infants; back blows and chest thrusts are safer and more effective. The Heimlich maneuver is used to aid older children and adults who are choking. To perform the Heimlich maneuver, stand behind the choking victim and wrap your arms around his waist. Make a fist with one hand and grasp the fist with the other hand. Place the thumb side of your fist on the upper abdomen and compress it with a quick inward and upward jerk, repeating several times if necessary. The pressure on the abdomen is transmitted to the lungs and forces the object up and out of the airway. It may take six to ten abdominal thrusts to dislodge a foreign object.

Swallowed Objects

Children often swallow small objects such as coins. These nearly always pass through the intestines and are eliminated in 3 to 5 days without causing any harm.

Occasionally, an object such as rock candy or a quarter may lodge in a child's esophagus, the tube running from the mouth to the stomach. An object stuck in a child's esophagus is less serious than one stuck in the windpipe. Excessive drooling, pain in the area where the object is stuck, and inability to swallow indicate that a foreign object may be stuck in the esophagus. Call your doctor, or take the child to the hospital.

Poisoning

The term poisoning refers to eating, drinking, inhaling, or touching something that may cause harm to the child. Symptoms may range from an upset stomach to a fatal injury.

Poison Control Centers

Consult your local hospital or yellow pages to find the phone number for the poison control center near you. Post the phone number near your telephone. Poison control centers specialize in up-to-date information on all kinds of poisonings and what to do about them. They also maintain a 24-hour physician consultation service. It is difficult for reference books and practicing physicians to keep up-to-date on every kind of harmful product. For this reason it is usually best to contact the poison control center before or in addition to contacting your own physician. When calling your poison control center have the following information readily available:

Name of the substance and the listed ingredients

Time of ingestion

Amount ingested

Age and weight of the child

Symptoms: coughing, vomiting, behavior changes

Your telephone number

Any other medical information about the child,
including any medications he has taken recently.

The following information, including the charts, is meant only as a general guide. Consult your physician or poison control center for the most up-to-date information on specific substances and what to do if your child swallows or comes into contact with them.

Poisonous Plants

There are approximately 300,000 plants in the United States and Canada; 525 are suspected to be poisonous. The effects of a poisonous plant may be only an uncomfortable irritation of the mouth and an upset stomach; with some plants, ingestion may be fatal. Fortunately the leaves of toxic plants have such an unpleasant taste that children seldom ingest large quantities of them.

If you think that a child has eaten part of a poisonous plant, check his hands and mouth for pieces. This will

Non-Harmful or Mildly Harmful Substances

Accidental ingestion of these substances does not usually require treatment. *Caution: This list is meant only as a general guide.* Consult your physician or poison control center for more information.

Antacids
Antibiotics (if only a few
    tablets or teaspoons)
Baby shampoos and lotions
Bath oil
Bath soap
Bubble bath
Calamine lotion
Candles
Caps (for toy pistols)
Chalk
Cigarettes[1]
Colognes
Cosmetics[2]
Crayons[3]
Dehumidifier packets
Deodorants
Deodorizers
Detergents[4]
Elmer's glue
Eye make-up
Fabric softeners
Fish bowl additives
Glues and pastes
Hand lotions and creams
Incense

Indelible markers
Ink
Laxatives
Lipstick
Lysol disinfectant (not toilet bowel
    cleaner)
Magic markers
Make-up
Matches
Mercury from broken thermometers
Modeling clay
Newspaper
Oral contraceptives
Pencil lead
Petroleum jelly (Vaseline)
Play-Doh
Putty and Silly Putty
Rouge
Shaving cream
Shampoos
Suntan preparations
Sweetening agents
Thyroid tablets
Vitamins with or without fluoride
Zinc oxide

1. Although one cigarette theoretically contains enough nicotine to be toxic, ingested tobacco is not easily absorbed from the intestines. The child frequently vomits and gets rid of much of the tobacco.

2. Most cosmetics are not generally harmful. However, permanent wave neutralizer and fingernail polish are extremely harmful. Even inhaling fumes from fingernail polish as it is being applied may be harmful to a child. Mouthwashes contain a large amount of alcohol and therefore can harm a child if ingested in large quantities.

3. Crayons labeled with AP, CP, or CS 130-46 designations are non-toxic.

4. Most household laundry detergents, cleansers, and dish detergents are not toxic. However, bleaches, ammonias and automatic dishwashing detergent granules and liquids may be highly toxic.

5. Iron in vitamins may be highly toxic if ingested in large amounts.

Source: *Handbook of Common Poisonings in Children*, 2d ed. (Evanston, Illinois: American Academy of Pediatrics, 1983.)

give you a good idea of whether or not the child actually ingested the plant. The most common and least serious symptoms of plant ingestion are swelling of the tongue, burning or blistering on the inside of the mouth and tongue, and vomiting, abdominal pain, and diarrhea. More serious but less common signs and symptoms of plant poisoning are an irregular and weak pulse, dizziness, convulsions, paralysis, unconsciousness, dry mouth, dilated pupils, intense sweating, shock, and not breathing. If you suspect that a child has eaten a harmful plant, contact the poison control center immediately for further instructions. Nearly all plant poisonings can be treated successfully by diluting the plant toxin by drinking large amounts of water and inducing vomiting.

What to Do for a Poisoning

If a child swallows a potentially harmful substance, encourage him to drink lots of water to dilute the poison. Then call your poison control center and follow the instructions you will be given over the phone.

How to induce vomiting. If the poison control center advises you to induce vomiting in the child, get out your poison prevention kit. Give the child one tablespoon (three teaspoons) of syrup of ipecac, followed by one to two eight-ounce glasses of water or non-carbonated fruit juice. Unless advised by the poison control center, do not give milk, as this may lessen the effectiveness of the ipecac. Have a large basin or pan nearby to try to collect the vomit so it can be inspected for the ingested poison, if necessary. Jostle or bounce your infant or child on your knee a few minutes as this mixes the ipecac with the stomach solution and hastens the vomiting. If vomiting does not occur within 20 minutes, repeat the dose of ipecac. Ipecac-induced vomiting is effective at least 90 percent of the time. Perform this ritual in the bathroom or kitchen since prolonged vomiting may occasionally follow a dose of ipecac. Observe the child for 45 minutes after he first vomits.

Non-Harmful House and Garden Plants

Accidental ingestion of these plants does not usually require treatment. *Caution: This list is meant only as a general guide. Consult your physician or poison control center for more information.*

African violet	Mother-in-law's tongue
Aralia	Pepperomia
Begonia	Piggyback plant
Boston fern	Pilea
Christmas cactus	Pink polka-dot plant
Coleus	Plectranthus
Dandelion	Prayer plant
Donkeytail	Rose
Dracaena	Rubber plant
Hawaii ti	Schefflera
Hen and chicks	Sensitive plant
Honeysuckle	Snapdragon
Hoya	Spider plant
Jade plant	Swedish ivy
Lipstick plant	Violet
Marigold	Wandering jew
Monkey plant	Weeping fig

Non-toxic berries

Acouba	High cranberry
Barberry	Mountain ash
Dogwood	Nindina

Sources: *Poisonous Plants of the United States and Canada* by J. Kingsbury (Englewood Cliffs, New Jersey: Prentice-Hall, 1964) and *Handbook of Common Poisonings in Children*, 2d ed. (Evanston, Illinois: American Academy of Pediatrics, 1983.)

Offer activated charcoal. After the vomiting has stopped, give the child a mixture of one to two tablespoons of activated charcoal in a glass of water. Stir this well and let the child take it through a straw. Use an empty soda can to disguise the solution. Activated charcoal absorbs some of the poison in the intestines, keeping it from entering the blood stream. Do not give the activated charcoal at the same time you give ipecac syrup because it may prevent the ipecac from working.

When not to induce vomiting. Do not induce vomiting before consulting with your poison control center. The ingested substance may not be harmful, and the child may not need treatment. Also, certain chemicals are more dangerous if vomited. They can cause damage to the lungs and the lining of the esophagus. Unless advised otherwise by the poison control center, do not induce vomiting when any of the following are ingested:

Petroleum products: gasoline, kerosene, benzene, turpentine

Polishes for furniture or cars

Strong corrosives such as lye, strong acids, drain cleaners

Cleaning products such as bleach, ammonia, toilet bowl cleaners.

Contact Poisons
When an irritating poison has come in contact with skin, remove any clothing that has the poison on it. (Be careful when doing this so that you don't spread the irritant to other areas of skin. Use a scissors if necessary. Leave the clothing on if you can't remove it safely.) Put the irritated area underneath the water faucet and rinse for several minutes. Wash with soap, but do not scrub the area right away since intense scrubbing may cause more of the poison to be absorbed into the skin.

Potentially Harmful House and Garden Plants

Accidental ingestion of these plants requires treatment. *Caution: This list is meant only as a general guide. Consult your physician or poison control center for more information.*

Amaryllis	Larkspur
Autumn crocus	Lily of the valley
Azalea	Mistletoe
Bird of paradise	Morning glory
Buttercup	Nightshade
Caster bean	Oleander
Croton	Philodendron
Daffodil	Poinsettia
Daphne	Poison ivy
Dieffenbachia	Poison oak
Elderberry	Poison sumac
Elephant ear	Poppy
English ivy	Rhododendron
Hemlock	Rhubarb leaves (stalks are edible)
Holly	Sweet pea (in large amounts)
Hyacinth	Tomato plants (stems and leaves)
Hydrangea	
Iris	Wild mushrooms
Jerusalem cherry	Wild tobacco
Jimson weed	Wisteria

Sources: *Poisonous Plants of the United States and Canada* by J. Kingsbury (Englewood Cliffs, New Jersey: Prentice-Hall, 1964) and *Handbook of Common Poisonings in Children*, 2d ed. (Evanston, Illinois: American Academy of Pediatrics, 1983.)

Splattering poisons in the eyes. Quickly wash an irritating substance out of the eye with tepid water. Hold the
eyelids open and flush the substance out of the eyes under a gentle stream from the water faucet or by splash-
ing water into the eye. Continue rinsing for at least five
minutes. Discourage the child from rubbing his eyes during and after the washing. If the irritating substance was
a strong acid or lye substance and/or the child continues
to experience intense eye pain, the cornea (the lining of
the eyeball) may have been damaged and should be examined and treated by a doctor.

Inhaled Poisons
Children may inhale the fumes of common household sol-
vents, cements, and glues. These contain acetone and
hydrocarbons which may be toxic to the lungs, kidneys,
and brain of the developing child. Use lacquers, varnishes,
glues, and cements in a well-ventilated room (preferably
outside), away from children. Nail polish and polish
removers, glues and lacquers for models, and varnishes
are the most common inhaled poisons in children.

Common Childhood Injuries

Head Injuries
There is a difference between a head injury and a brain
injury. Because the skull acts as a protective helmet for
the brain, most blows to the head injure only the scalp
tissues and bones but not the underlying brain. The scalp
is very richly supplied with blood vessels. For this reason, even a small wound on the head bleeds profusely.
When any tissue rich in blood vessels, such as a scalp,
is suddenly compressed between two hard objects (e.g.,
the floor and the skull) small blood vessels within the scalp
are easily broken, resulting in the characteristic "goose-
egg." Don't be alarmed at the quick appearance and large
size of these bumps after a blow to the skull. With ice
packs and pressure they go down very quickly. Because

of the rich blood supply, scalp wounds do not become infected as easily as do wounds to other parts of the body.
Most goose-eggs are a sign of injury only to the scalp tissue and not to the underlying brain.

The two main concerns in head injuries are bleeding
and concussion. When the small blood vessels between
the skull and the brain have been broken, bleeding occurs between the brain and the skull. Because the skull
is like a rigid helmet, any bleeding between the skull and
the brain compresses the brain. A blow to the head may
also shake the brain, resulting in an injury called a concussion. Pressure upon the brain from bleeding or from
the swelling associated with a concussion produces symptoms of head injury.

What to Do for a Head Injury

If your child has a cut or scrape on the scalp, apply ice
and pressure for 20 minutes. This will reduce the size of
the goose-egg. If the child is unconscious but breathing
normally and his color is good (lips are not blue), lay the
child down on a flat surface and call the rescue squad for
transportation to the local hospital. If there is reason to
suspect a neck injury, do not move the child until experts
in the transportation of children with head and neck injuries arrive. If the child is not breathing, or convulsions
occur, follow the guidelines in the sections on CPR (pages
204-207) and convulsions (pages 229-230).

Period of observation.   If the child is alert and conscious,
is walking, talking, and resumes play, administer the usual
parental sympathy and begin a period of observation. If
pressure is going to develop in the brain, either from bleeding or from swelling, the symptoms may not appear for
several hours. Watch for the following signs.

Change in the level of alertness. Is the child talking well, responding to simple questions? Does he seem
aware of who he is and where he is? It is usual for the
child to fall asleep following any injury since sleep is a

normal state of refuge for an upset child. Let your child
sleep, but awaken him every two hours. During his sleep
observe him for a change in color or breathing patterns.
If over the next six to eight hours your child continues
to be as alert and active as he was prior to the injury, then
an underlying brain injury is unlikely.

Watch the eyes. The eyes are the mirror of the brain,
as well as the soul, especially in the event of a head injury. If your child looks at you straight in the eye with
the usual bright penetrating look so typical of children,
underlying brain injury is unlikely. Observe the child's
pupils. Are they both the same size? Check his vision. Hold
up your hand and ask him how many fingers he sees. Point
to known objects across the room and ask him to name
them. Cover one eye at a time. Does he complain of seeing double? Crossed eyes, seeing double, blurred vision,
and one pupil being much larger than the other are all
signs of a possible brain injury.

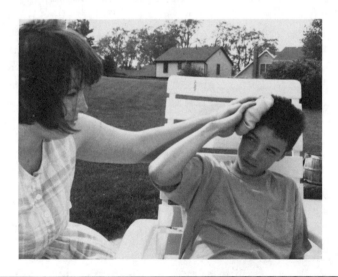

Ice and pressure will help reduce the swelling of a head injury.
A period of observation will determine if the injury is serious.

Walking style. Observe the child's walking style. If it is steady and the same as it was prior to the injury, this is a good sign. If the child is persistently off-balance, wobbly, or showing weakness in one arm or leg, an underlying brain injury may be present. In the child who is not yet walking, observe sitting-up and crawling motions. Are they the same as before the injury?

Persistent vomiting. Children will often vomit once or twice after a head injury, even if there is no underlying brain injury. If the vomiting persists or begins again several hours after the injury occurs, this is cause for concern. It is wise to feed only clear fluids for a few hours after a head injury, in case vomiting occurs.

Headaches. These are to be expected after a head injury, but they usually subside within a few hours. If headaches increase in severity, be concerned. Do not give aspirin for a headache as it may aggravate bleeding. Use acetaminophen instead.

When to call your doctor. Unless the child obviously has a brain injury (abnormalities in walking, talking, and vision), it is important that you observe the child for several hours before calling your doctor. Your doctor will ask you all of the above questions anyway and will rely heavily on your observations in deciding whether this is simply a scalp injury or if there is an underlying brain injury. After the period of observation, check with your doctor, who may instruct you to watch for additional signs. Depending on the severity of the injury your doctor may advise you that it is not necessary to awaken your child during the night. If there is any persistent change in your child's behavior following a head injury, call your doctor.

Skull x-rays. Most children with head injuries do not need skull x-rays. Generally, a child who has not had any of the previous concerning symptoms does not require a skull x-ray. A period of observation and a medical examination is usually more useful than an x-ray. A skull fracture in itself is not harmful if there is no injury to the brain. A longer period of observation is more valuable than an immediate skull x-ray in the medical assessment of a child with head injuries. A negative skull x-ray may lull one into a false sense of security when, in fact, there is an underlying brain injury. A CAT scan, a series of cross-sectional x-rays of the brain, is often performed in the emergency room following a severe injury to the head. CAT scans give a lot of information about whether there is bleeding or swelling of the brain. Depending on the severity and the course of the head injury, your doctor may order this test.

Nose Injuries

The nose is beautifully designed to function as a shock absorber, so that blows to the face do not injure the head. When the nose collides with a hard surface (e.g., your child runs into a pole, falls flat on his face, or is hit by a flying fist) the nose flattens as the thin nasal bones are pushed out to each side. If these bones did not give easily in response to trauma, the pressure of the blow would be transmitted to the internal structures of the head.

When the nose gets banged up, apply an ice pack for at least a half hour. Press the ice pack on the bulged-out swollen areas on each side of the nose, just below the nasal corner of the eyes.

When to seek medical attention. Because they are effective shock absorbers, the nasal bones fracture very easily, but they also usually reset themselves very easily within a couple of weeks after the injury. After you have applied ice and pressure for at least half an hour, check your child's nose to see if you need to seek medical attention. Look for cosmetic distortion of the nasal bones (the nose is angled to one side). Check for obstruction of breathing by gently compressing one nostril and then the other. If either cosmetic distortion or obstruction of air flow is present, seek medical attention.

Nosebleeds. Some children have nosebleeds frequently. They are usually due to nose-picking and damage to the small blood vessels lining the inside of the nose. Nosebleeds are common during allergy season due to increased nose picking and scratching. Nosebleeds are also common in the winter, when the low humidity of central heating dries out and irritates the lining of the nose. This problem is usually alleviated by increasing the humidity in the child's bedroom when the central heating is in use. The crust around the opening to the nose can be softened by applying petroleum jelly with a cotton-tipped applicator.

How to stop a nosebleed. Sit the child on a chair, leaning slightly forward. Apply pressure by pinching the nostrils together for at least ten minutes without releasing the pressure. Many nosebleeds originate in the blood vessels lining the middle bone of the nose, called the nasal septum. To apply pressure to these vessels insert a twisted piece of wet cotton into the bleeding nostril. This piece of cotton should fit snugly and be large enough to fill two-thirds of the nasal opening. The cotton transmits the pressure from the pinched nostrils to the nasal septum. Pressure may also be applied to the major vessels supplying the nose; these are located where the upper lip joins the gum, just below the nostrils. Place a piece of wet cotton underneath the upper lip and apply pressure with two fingers upward in the direction of the nostrils, or on the outside of the lip just below the nostrils.

The child should sit upright and not lie down. This prevents blood from dripping into his throat. Persistent swallowing of blood may cause a child to feel nauseated and to vomit the blood. After the nosebleed has been controlled, discourage the child from sniffing or sneezing through his nose, as this may dislodge the clot and cause the bleeding to start again. Have him keep his mouth open in case he needs to sneeze or cough through his mouth. Once the bleeding stops, leave the piece of cotton lodged in the nostril for 12 to 24 hours to allow a clot to form over the blood vessel—particularly if the child suffers from frequent nosebleeds. Remove the cotton plug gently in order not to dislodge the clot and cause bleeding to recur.

If the nosebleed continues despite the above measures, consult your doctor or take the child to the hospital. The bleed may require nasal packing or cauterization (drying up) of the blood vessel.

Discourage your child from picking his nose. Children seldom admit to picking their nose. To elicit a confession, try the following trick: ask your child "Which finger do you use to pick your nose?" Before the child has time to disavow that he picks his nose, he will usually extend the telltale forefinger. Cut his fingernails very short and explain to your child how picking is damaging his nose.

Foreign objects in the nose. Children four years and younger often place small objects such as beans or peas into their nose. Children often do not complain of an object in their nose, but you may suspect this if there is a very foul-smelling discharge from one nostril. To remove foreign objects from the nose, try the following:

If you can see the object, attempt to remove it with blunt-end tweezers.

If the object is lodged far back into the nose, compress the unblocked nostril and encourage the child to sneeze with his mouth closed. Often this will dislodge the foreign object.

If the object is water-soluble, such as a piece of candy, take the child into the shower and get a lot of steam up the nose. Or squirt some saltwater nose drops up into the nose to soften the object and reduce its size.

If the object is still lodged far back in the nose and you are unable to remove it with the above measures, take the child to the hospital where a doctor can remove the object with a special instrument. Do not allow your child to lie on his back or fall asleep with a foreign object in his nose since it may be aspirated into the lungs.

Fractures, Sprains, Strains, and Contusions

The unique structures around children's joints make them prone to types of injuries seldom seen in adults. Near the end of each bone, children have soft areas called growth plates. This is the area of the bone which grows longer as the child grows. Because these growth plates are weaker than the ligaments which hold one bone to another, a sudden force applied to the bone may cause the growth plate to separate. This is called a growth plate fracture and is unique to children's bones until they have attained full growth, at approximately 18 years of age. If a growth plate injury is not properly diagnosed and treated, growth of the bone may be disturbed and shortening of the affected limb may result. The same type of injury in an adult would result in a torn ligament or a sprained ankle. The end of the bone is the weakest part of a child's joint; in an adult, the ligaments and supporting tissues around the joint are the weakest point. This is why children tend to break bones more easily than adults.

When deciding whether to seek medical attention for a bone or joint injury, look for the following:

Swelling

Pain

Limitation of motion

Point tenderness.

Ask the child to point to the area of pain. If he points to the area with one finger and can pinpoint the pain in a small area the size of a quarter, there probably is an underlying fracture. Children usually hold an injured limb still, in a position that provides maximum pain avoidance. For example, if a child has an injury to his elbow, he may hold the affected arm flexed against his body with his other hand, as if making his own sling. If you suspect a fracture, take your child to the hospital.

Toddler fractures are a common, non-serious fracture to the midshaft of the long bone of the legs. They usually occur during the frequent falls of the beginning walker. Sometimes these go undiagnosed and untreated and only show up years later as an old healed fracture on an x-ray taken for some other injury. Limping and unwillingness to bear weight on the affected limb are the usual signs of toddler fractures; medical attention should be obtained. A limp which lasts longer than 24 hours always warrants medical attention, mainly to be sure there is no injury to the hip joint.

A **contusion** is a bruise that does not break the skin. It happens when the body is struck, such as during a fall or a bump. This results in pain and swelling at the site of the injury. The pain is worsened when the muscle is used. Contusions usually subside within a day or two. Elevate the area and apply ice.

Muscle strains are common when a child begins a new sport or a new exercise routine and uses muscles that

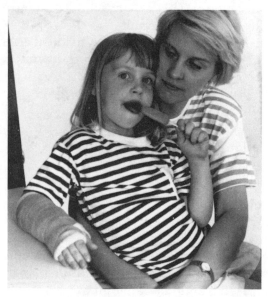

A hug and a treat follow a trip to
the emergency room for a broken arm.

have not previously been conditioned. Sometimes a severe muscle strain may be associated with bleeding within the muscle, causing stiffness and pain on movement. Heat, massage, and elevation usually relieve the pain and allow the muscle to heal quickly. Muscle strains during sports can be minimized by encouraging your child to stretch the muscles gently and warm up before practices or games.

First Aid for Strains, Sprains, and Fractures

What to do for common orthopedic injuries is summed up in the acronym ICES: ice, compression, elevation, and support. All four of these treatments are designed to slow down continued bleeding within the joint or muscle and thus shorten the recovery time.

Ice should be applied to any muscle, bone, or joint injury that is swollen. Ice decreases muscle spasms, pain, bleeding, and swelling. Put crushed ice in a cloth, bag, or towel and apply it to the site of injury for at least 20 minutes. Do not apply ice directly to the skin as this may cause frostbite. Unless advised by your doctor, do not apply heat to any orthopedic injury for the first 48 hours, as this will increase bleeding and swelling. Heat is often used a few days after the injury to help resolve the bleeding in the joint and increase the blood supply in the area to enhance healing.

Compression also helps to minimize swelling. Using an elastic bandage, wrap the affected joint beginning at the point farthest away from the heart. The bandage should be just snug enough to insert one finger beneath it. If the fingers or toes beyond the bandage begin to swell, turn blue, or feel numb, the bandage is too tight.

Elevate the affected limb about six inches using a pillow. If the ankle is injured also place a pillow under the back of the knee to allow the child to flex the leg slightly. If the arm or wrist is injured, let the child sleep on his back or side with the affected arm elevated on a pillow.

Support the affected limb with crutches, a cane, or a sling to prevent unnecessary motion or weight-bearing.

When a muscle is not used for more than three or four days, it becomes weakened. Rehabilitation is very important after a muscle or joint injury. When the child does begin to use the muscle again, he should be given exercises to gradually rebuild its strength. Check with your doctor for specific instructions. Doing too much too soon with a rested muscle may result in another injury.

Pulled Elbow

You're walking along the sidewalk with your two-year-old who has a habit of darting away from you out into the street. Sure enough, there he goes, and your first instinct is to grab his arm and jerk him back to you, to keep him out of the oncoming traffic. A few minutes later, he's complaining that his arm hurts; it hangs limply at his side and he refuses to use it. Or he may hold it bent across his chest with his other arm.

This injury is called a pulled elbow, and it happens when the forearm bone slips out of the elbow joint. Sometimes the bone slips back into place easily, and the child will be free of pain and use his arm normally again. Otherwise, it requires medical attention. Take the child to your doctor or to a hospital emergency room where a physician can put the bone back in its proper location by flexing and twisting the arm until the elbow pops back into place. Once the elbow is back in place, it is necessary to place the child's arm in a sling for two days to allow the stretched ligaments to heal. Pulled elbows can be avoided. Don't jerk your child's arm suddenly when he tries to pull away. Do not try too pick up a child or swing him by only one arm.

Eye Injuries

When a foreign object—a speck of dust, a tiny piece of metal—gets stuck in a child's eye, there will be a burning sensation, excessive tearing, overall redness, and increased prominence of the blood vessels in the whites of the eye. Besides causing pain, foreign bodies can scratch the surface of the eye and therefore should be removed as soon as possible.

To remove a foreign object from a child's eye, gently pull down the lower lid and encourage the child to open his eyes very wide as you irrigate it with a gentle stream from a pitcher of water. If the stream of water does not remove the foreign body, try to locate the object and determine whether it is on the eyeball itself or is caught underneath the upper or lower eyelid. Pull down the lower lid to see if the object is there. If you suspect it is under the upper eyelid, tell the child to look down, and then pull the upper eyelid down over the lower eyelid. The lashes of the lower eyelid may dislodge the foreign body from beneath the upper eyelid.

If this method is unsuccessful, tell the child to look down, and then grasp the upper eyelashes with your thumb and index finger and gently pull the lid away from the eyeball. Place a cotton-tipped applicator horizontally along the center of the upper lid. Pull the lid forward and upward thereby causing it to fold back over the applicator, exposing the underside. Using a wisp of moist cotton or the edge of a clean moist handkerchief, flick the foreign body from the surface of the eyelid.

Do not attempt to remove a foreign body from the surface of the eyeball. This should be done by a doctor. Never use dry tissue or cotton near the eye as this may scratch the eyeball.

When to call your doctor.   If you have removed the foreign body from the eyelid and the child has no pain in his eyeball, you may safely assume there has been no injury to the eyeball. If the eye still hurts, the foreign body may not have been completely removed or the eyeball has been scratched. In this case you should call your doctor. The doctor will examine the eyeball. If it has been scratched, he may prescribe an antibiotic ointment to prevent infection. Slivers of metal or other objects imbedded in the eye should be removed only by an eye doctor.

Chemical irritations. Irritating substances may splash into the eye. Pour a glass of water into the child's eye or have him hold his eye under a gentle stream of water from the faucet or immerse his eye in a pan of water. Because chemical irritations are extremely painful, a child may be unwilling to open his eyes to do this. You may have to hold his eyelid open while you are irrigating the eye. Water irrigation should continue for at least 10 minutes, and then you should call your doctor. It is best to cover both eyes with a blindfold, as this slows down the eye movements which may aggravate both the pain and the injury. Explain why you are covering his eyes and provide lots of emotional support; children frighten easily when their eyes are covered.

Burns

Burns are one of the most common and most painful childhood injuries. First-degree burns, such as sunburns, usually do not require extensive treatment. A second-degree burn has blisters. A third-degree burn is deep and has an area of charred or white skin. Complications from burns include infection, loss of body fluids from the burned area, scarring, and impairment of function.

To treat a burn, immediately submerge the area in cold water for at least twenty minutes. Besides alleviating pain, this cools the skin and lessens tissue damage. Do not use ice packs or bare ice cubes on burns as this may increase tissue damage. Cover the burned area with a clean cloth; do not apply oils or butter. If there are several blisters or the skin is charred or white, call your doctor or take the child to the hospital.

The long-term treatment of burns is aimed at alleviating pain, preventing infection, improving cosmetic healing, and preventing contractures (shortening of the burned tissue as it heals). Follow your physician's advice. The usual steps for treatment of burns start with washing the burned area at least twice a day under a stream of water, such as the tap or the shower, and blotting it dry with a clean towel. In addition to cleansing the area, the jet of water removes dead tissue. Do not break blisters without your doctor's advice; blisters are nature's "dressings."

Keep the burn covered with an ointment such as Silvadene (by prescription), which promotes healing and lessens infections. Your doctor will instruct you on how to apply a burn dressing and how frequently to change it; usually morning and night changes are sufficient.

If the burn is over a joint or a place where the body flexes, such as the palm of the hand or the joints of the fingers, it is important to stretch the burned area to avoid contracture of the tissue as it heals. Do this for at least a minute or two ten times a day.

Periodically, during the healing of the burn, it may be necessary for you or your doctor to remove some of the burned tissue in order to minimize infection as the burn is healing. This is called debridement. Follow your doctor's advice and instructions.

Pain relief. Burns are extremely painful, at least for the first few hours. Cold water and analgesics are the best pain relievers.

Depending on the severity, a properly treated burn usually heals well within two weeks. With careful medical follow-up, frequent dressing changes, application of burn ointment, and debridement, most childhood burns will heal completely, without noticeable scarring.

Convulsions

Convulsions are extremely scary for both children and parents. They occur when the electrical circuits of the brain discharge abnormally. Convulsions have a wide range of severity, varying from occasional twitching of one

arm to a total body convulsion, called a grand mal sei-
zure. This is characterized by the jerking of all the muscles of the body, especially the extremities, falling and
writhing on the ground, rolling back of the eyes, profuse
salivation, and, often, temporary loss of consciousness.

Emergency treatment of a convulsion is aimed at getting the child to resume normal breathing in order to prevent oxygen deprivation to the brain. If your child has a
severe convulsion, place him on the floor, in the prone
position (stomach down) with his head turned to one side.
This allows gravity to drain the secretions in his throat.

Keep him away from furniture and walls that he could
strike while thrashing. If the child's lips are not blue during the convulsion and he seems to be breathing, it is unlikely that the convulsion will cause the child any harm.
If the child is blue and not breathing, call the paramedics
immediately and begin mouth-to-mouth breathing (see
pages 204-205). It is important to give the child enough
air and oxygen, since lowered amounts of oxygen going
to the brain will worsen the convulsion.

Most convulsions in children under five are due to sudden high fever, although the fever may have previously
gone unnoticed. If a child has a febrile convulsion reduce
the fever as quickly as possible. Undress your child completely, place cool towels over him, and cool his environment. (See Chapter Four for more suggestions on lowering
a fever.) Febrile convulsions usually stop within seconds,
as soon as the fever declines. After the convulsion subsides consult your doctor for further advice and medical
attention.

Cuts and Scratches

When a child gets a cut, the first thing to do is stop the
bleeding. Apply pressure with gauze or a clean cloth until the bleeding stops, usually around ten minutes. If your
child has cut a major blood vessel, apply a pressure bandage for at least twenty minutes. A pressure bandage is

made by placing a pad of sterile gauze or a clean cloth directly over the wound and taping and holding it in place for at least twenty minutes. Even if the blood soaks through the cloth, do not remove the first cloth since that could dislodge the clot that helps close the wound. Add more layers of gauze or cloth on top of the first.

Maintain steady pressure on the center of the bandage, keeping the pad firmly in place as you wrap more gauze over the pad. Ice packs may help stop the bleeding and lessen the swelling, but never apply ice directly to a bare wound as this may further damage the tissue.

After the bleeding has stopped, rinse off the wound with cool water from the faucet or shower to assess whether or not it will need stitches. Cleanse the wound with soap and water; a stream of water from the faucet or shower will help wash out the dirt.

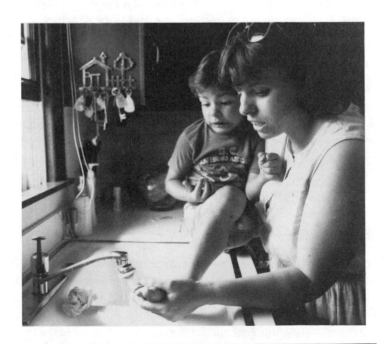

Running water removes dirt from a cut.

Apply a moist gauze pad to the wound to keep the edges from drying out. Saturate the gauze with antibiotic ointment. Elevate the wound area so that it is higher than the level of the heart. This helps control bleeding and swelling. Call your doctor or take the child to the hospital if you need further advice as to whether stitches or a special type of bandage will be needed. If your child has had his initial series of five tetanus shots, a tetanus booster is needed only once every ten years.

Abrasions

Abrasions (scratches) result when the outer layers of skin are scraped off. They do not usually need stitches, but they are often very painful. They can easily become infected because of the damage to the outer layer of skin and the dirt that may be imbedded in the wound. Clean all debris such as sand, dirt, or pieces of glass from the wound. Usually a jet of cool water and light rubbing with gauze will cleanse the wound. Use antiseptic soap such as Hibiclens. Do not use cleansing solutions such as alcohol which burn and sting. Abrasions are often more painful than cuts since a larger area of the skin is damaged and the nerve fibers are exposed. Keep the wound covered with a dressing and antibiotic ointment. If the abrasion is on the face or another exposed area, avoid prolonged exposure of the wound to bright sunlight for four to six months; sunburn will increase the scarring and produce irregular skin pigmentation as the abrasion is healing.

Insect Stings

Insect stings become very painful and swollen because of the stinger and the injected venom. Bees leave their stinger and its attached venom sack in the wound. Scrape away the protruding poison sack with a sharp knife before removing the rest of the stinger. Squeezing the sack with tweezers will only force more venom into the skin. Wasp stingers do not have an attached venom sack. After removing the stinger, apply ice to the sting site; this slows down the spread of the venom and eases the pain.

The main danger with insect stings is an allergic reaction to the venom. Most stings produce localized pain and swelling. This does not harm the child and subsides within a day; you need to treat it only with ice and elevation. However, some children have allergic reactions to insect stings. If there is swelling of the hands, eyelids, and eyes, or if the child is wheezing and having breathing difficulties, take him immediately to the hospital, as these type of allergic reactions tend to become rapidly more severe.

If your child has previously had an allergic reaction to an insect sting and gets stung again, apply a tourniquet above the site of the sting, if it occurs on the arm or leg. The tourniquet should be just tight enough to allow you to slip your index finger under it. Apply ice to the sting site and elevate the affected limb. Take the child to the hospital emergency room immediately, even if you have to sit in the waiting room to see if a severe allergic reaction occurs.

If your child has had repeated severe allergic reactions to stinging insects, allergy shots can be very effective in desensitizing the child to the venom.

If you are traveling and your child has a history of reactions to insect stings, ask your doctor for an emergency insect sting kit (including adrenalin) and directions on how to use it. These are very valuable when traveling a long distance away from medical facilities such as on a camping trip.

During your years of active parenting, you will spend lots of time caring for your child's illnesses and "ouchies." Remember that you are taking care of the whole child, not just a disease or an injury. When he is hurting, he is probably also frightened and upset. Your tender care helps him to master his feelings. It is also a sign of your love.

INDEX

Ipecac syrup, 33, 175
Iron, 10

Jaundice in newborns, 35-39
  frequent breastfeeding prevents,
    37-38

Lactase insufficiency, 112
Lactobacillus bifidus, 8
Laxatives, 33
Lethargy, 22
Lice, 153-54
Life jackets, 198

Mattresses, crib, 180
Measles, 142-43
  complications, 143
  contagiousness, 142
  rash, 142
  vaccine, 14, 15, 143
Measles, German
  See Rubella
Medicine
  for colds, 68-69
  expiration date, 27
  giving, 27-30
  to keep on hand, 31-33
  for skin problems, 160
  spitting up, 28
  storing safely, 175
Meningism, 151
Meningitis, 150-51
Milia, 41
MMR vaccine, 14, 15
  reactions to, 18
Mouth-to-mouth resuscitation, 204-5
Mumps, 143-44
  vaccine, 14, 15, 144
Muscle strains, 224-25
  treating, 225-26

Night light, 176
Nipples, sore, 41
Nose
  broken, 220
  cleaning out infant's, 65
  foreign object in, 222
  teaching child to blow, 67
Nose drops, 33, 69
  for sinus infections, 91
Nosebleeds, 221-22
Nurseries, church, 10-11
Nutrition, 7-10
  during illness, 26

Otitis media
  See Ear, middle, infections
Otitis media, serous, 79-80
Otitis externa, 87

Pain relievers, 26-27
Paint, leaded, 175, 180
Parenting style, 1-4, 21-22
Peaked, defined, 22
Pertussis, 74
Pertussis vaccine, 14-16
  reactions to, 17-18
Pets, 127-28
Pharyngitis
  See Sore throat
Phototherapy, 39
Physician, 4-5, 12
Pinworms, 151-53
Plants, poisonous, 178, 210, 215
Playground equipment, 178
Playpens, 186
Pneumonia, 100-2
Poison control center, 175, 209-10
Poison ivy, 162-63
Poison oak, 162-63
Poison prevention kit, 175
Poisoning, 209-16
  contact poisons, 214
  in the eye, 216
  inhaled, 216
  non-harmful substances, 211, 213
  what to do, 212, 214
Polio vaccine, 14, 15
  in breastfed baby, 18
  reactions to, 18
Pool safety, 179, 196-98
Prickly heat, 41-42
Product Safety, Department of
  (Canada), 179, 189
Prolactin, 3
Pulse, checking, 206
Pyloric stenosis, 117-18
Pyrogens, 50

Rashes
  in babies, 41-45
  chicken pox, 137-38
  contact dermatitis, 161-62
  diaper, 43-45
  eczema, 159
  hives, 163
  impetigo, 164
  measles, 142
  ringworm, 168

THE GROWING FAMILY SERIES

The better you know your children, the more you will enjoy them— and you will find it easier to meet the challenges of parenting. The books in La Leche League's Growing Family Series are written to help parents develop a close relationship with their children from birth onward.

NIGHTTIME PARENTING
by William Sears, MD
Dr. Sears explains how babies sleep differently than adults, how sharing sleep can help the whole family sleep better, and how parents can lower the risk of Sudden Infant Death Syndrome. He also discusses night-waking, bedtime rituals, sleep disorders, and why babies should not be left to ''cry it out.'' **No. 276, softcover, 204 pages, $7.95**

THE FUSSY BABY
by William Sears, MD
This book has lots of suggestions for coping with fussy, high-need babies and toddlers, including ''back to the womb'' techniques for newborns and discipline methods for young children. Chapters on coping with colic, feeding, fathering, soothing, and avoiding maternal burnout include practical tips and reassurance. **No. 269, softcover, 207 pages, $7.95**

BECOMING A FATHER
by William Sears, MD
Written especially for fathers, this book addresses the joys and stresses of parenthood from the male perspective. There are practical tips on everything from how to hold and comfort tiny babies to helping children participate in organized sports. Dr. Sears also provides a guide to understanding the emotions of new mothers and the effects of children upon a marriage. **No. 266, softcover, 242 pages, $7.95**

GROWING TOGETHER
by William Sears, MD
The first year of life is an important one. Babies learn about their world, and parents learn about their babies. This book answers the ''What-will-my-baby-do-when?'' questions and tells parents how they can enhance their baby's development by their responsiveness. More than 150 black-and-white photos and 16 pages of color photos illustrate the growth of motor, language, social, and cognitive skills. **No. 273, softcover, 245 pages, $14.50**

Order from: La Leche League International, P. O. Box 1209, Franklin Park, IL 60131–8209 U.S.A. In Canada, send orders to LLLI Canadian Office, Williamsburg, Ontario K0C 2H0. (Please include $2.50 shipping and handling for one book; $3.50 for two or three books; $4.25 for four books. In California and Illinois, please add sales tax.)

LA LECHE LEAGUE MEMBERSHIP

La Leche League was founded in 1956 by seven women who had learned about successful breastfeeding while nursing their own babies. They wanted to share the information with other mothers. Now over 9,000 League Leaders and 3,500 League Groups carry on that legacy. League Leaders are always willing to answer questions about breastfeeding and mothering and are available by phone for help with breastfeeding problems. League Groups meet monthly in communities all over the world to share breastfeeding information and mothering experiences.

When you join La Leche League your annual membership fee of $25.00 brings you six bimonthly issues of NEW BEGINNINGS, a magazine filled with stories, tips, and inspiration from other breastfeeding families. Members receive our LLLI Catalogues by mail, and they are entitled to a 10 percent discount on purchases from LLLI's wide variety of outstanding books and publications on breastfeeding, childbirth, nutrition, and parenting. The Catalogue includes other products as well, among them the Original Dr. Sears Baby Sling.

Return this form to La Leche League International, P. O. Box 1209, Franklin Park, IL 60131–8209 U. S. A.

_____ I'd like to join La Leche League International. Enclosed is my annual membership fee of $25.00.

_____ In addition, I am enclosing a tax-deductible donation of $_____ to support the work of La Leche League.

_____ Please send me La Leche League's FREE Catalogue.

Name

Address

City

State/Province   Zip/Postal code   Country